WHY DOES GOD ALLOW BAD THINGS TO HAPPEN TO GOOD PEOPLE?

... And 5 Other Important Beliefs About God.

By Katie Storm

Part of the Big Ideas for Baby Christians Series

CONTENTS

INTRODUCTION

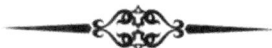

---◆◆◆---

by Katie Storm

Welcome to "Why Does God Allow Bad Things to Happen to Good People?"

This book is part of an ongoing series of books that explore some of the most profound questions about faith and suffering. Each Volume is guided by six key beliefs about God, all rooted in biblical teachings.

You may wonder why we chose such a challenging title for this book. It reflects a question many of us grapple with: Why do bad things happen to good people? This pivotal question is addressed in Chapter 1, where I encourage you to reflect deeply on the insights provided.

The material in this book has its origins in my earlier work, "Big Ideas for Baby Christians." I collaborated with my podcast partner, Terence. Together, we expanded on these ideas through our engaging podcast. Each Chapter in this book follows a similar format, offering commentary, along with study guides to help deepen your understanding.

Here are the six beliefs about God that we'll explore together in this book:

Chapter 1: Why Does God Allow Bad Things to Happen to Good People?

Chapter 2: How does God Use the Problems and Struggles in My Life for His Ultimate Good, and Mine?

Chapter 3: Why God Always Love You Unconditionally?

Chapter 4: The 3 Reasons God is Always With You and Will Never Leave You.

Chapter 5: Why God Wants You to Be Happy and Health and Excited About Living!

Chapter 6: Here is Actual Proof That God Does Not Want You to Be Fat, Sick, Depressed, or Unhappy. How Do You Know for Sure That God Has Your Best Interest in Mind? Here is the Proof!

As you read through each Chapter, consider listening to the corresponding Podcast audio, which can enhance your understanding of these concepts.

Don't miss Chapter 7, which tackles the vital question: Is Jesus God? This chapter is crucial for anyone seeking to understand the foundations of their faith.

At the end, you'll also find an invitation to learn more about our Membership.

Thank you for joining us on this journey. I hope you find inspiration, clarity, and strength as we explore these beliefs together. If you have any questions along the way, please feel free to reach out.

Let's begin!

CHAPTER ONE

BELIEF #1

Why does God allow bad things to happen to good people?

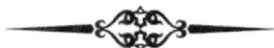

—✦—

CHAPTER ONE / BELIEF #1 – TABLE OF CONTENTS

BELIEF #1

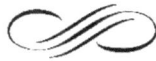

Why does God allow bad things to happen to good people?

This is one of the most challenging questions that people of faith often wrestle with. It's a question that has been asked for centuries and one that doesn't have a simple, straightforward answer. However, the Bible does offer insights that can help us understand God's perspective on suffering, and while it may not answer all our questions, it can provide comfort and guidance as we navigate through life's difficulties.

First, it's important to recognize that suffering is a part of the human experience. **The Bible doesn't shy away from this reality. In fact, Jesus himself said,** "In this godless world you will continue to experience difficulties. But take heart! I've conquered the world" (John 16:33, MSG). Jesus acknowledges that we will face challenges and hardships in this life. The presence of suffering doesn't mean that God is absent or that He doesn't care. Instead, it's a reminder that we live in a broken world where pain and suffering are part of our reality.

One reason God allows suffering is that it can help us grow and develop as individuals. The Bible often compares the process of spiritual growth to that of refining precious metals. In the book of James, we read, "Consider it a sheer gift, friends, when tests and challenges come at you from all sides. You know that under pressure, your faith-life is forced into the open and shows its true colors" (James 1:2-3, MSG). Trials and difficulties can reveal what's truly in our hearts and push us to rely more on God. They can also build our character, making us stronger and more resilient in our faith.

Another important aspect to consider is the concept of free will. God created humans with the ability to choose, and with that choice comes the possibility of choosing actions that lead to suffering. Some of the bad things that happen to good people are a result of the wrong choices made by others. **This doesn't mean that God is indifferent to our suffering.** In fact, the Bible tells us that God is deeply moved by our pain. "The Lord is close to the brokenhearted; he rescues those whose spirits are crushed" (Psalm 34:18, MSG). God is not distant or detached; He is near to those who are hurting and offers comfort and hope in the midst of their pain.

One of the most difficult aspects of suffering is when it seems completely unjust, when bad things happen to people who appear to be doing everything right. The Bible acknowledges this paradox, and we see it in the story of Job. Job was a man described as "blameless and upright," yet he faced unimaginable suffering. The book of Job doesn't offer a neat answer to why he suffered, **but it does show that suffering isn't always a direct result of a person's actions.** Sometimes, there is a mystery to suffering that we cannot fully comprehend.

However, the story of Job also reveals a crucial truth: God is sovereign, and His ways are beyond our understanding. When Job questioned God about his suffering, God responded by reminding Job of His power and wisdom in creation. Job ultimately recognized that he couldn't fully grasp God's purposes but chose to trust Him anyway. This teaches us that while we may not understand why we suffer, we can trust that **God has a greater plan that is beyond our limited perspective.**

Finally, the Bible gives us hope that suffering is not the end of the story. In Romans 8:18, we read, "That's why I don't think there's any comparison between the present hard times and the coming good times" (MSG). For those who trust in God, there is a promise of future restoration and joy that far outweighs the pain of this life. This doesn't minimize our suffering, but it gives us a perspective of hope, knowing that **God will one day make all things right.**

In conclusion, while the question of why God allows bad things to happen to good people is complex, the Bible offers insights that can help us navigate through it. Suffering is a part of life in a broken world, but **it can also be a tool for growth and a reminder of our need for God.** Free will plays a role in the suffering we experience, but God is always near to comfort us. Ultimately, while we may not fully understand the reasons for our suffering, we can trust in God's sovereignty and hold on to the hope of a future where all wrongs are made right.

THE PODCAST TRANSCRIPT

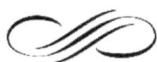

TERENCE: Okay, so have you ever had one of those days or weeks or months even where something bad happens and you just think, why me?

KATIE: It's certainly a question that has resonated with people for centuries,

TERENCE: Like the age old question, right? Why do bad things happen to good people?

KATIE: Right?

TERENCE: And that's what we're diving into today with this deep dive, going through some excerpts from a text that really digs into this idea of faith and suffering.

KATIE: And it's a question that continues to be relevant, I think, because it reflects a very deep human need to find meaning, especially in the face of hardship.

TERENCE: Totally. So where do we even begin with something as big as this?

KATIE: Well, what I find interesting about this particular text is that it doesn't shy away from the reality of suffering. It doesn't offer these simplistic answers or try to sugarcoat the very real struggles that people face. It's kind of refreshing, right? Like, yeah, life is tough sometimes. No kidding.

TERENCE: Exactly. It acknowledges that life can be messy and painful at times, and that those experiences are a part of the human condition.

KATIE: And then it goes a step further, doesn't it? It tackles this idea that just because you're suffering doesn't mean you've done something wrong. Like it's not punishment from God, right?

TERENCE: Right. It challenges that very common misconception. It's not about God being absent or not caring, but rather it uses this idea of a broken world to explain why suffering exists

KATIE: Broken world. Okay, so what does that even mean? Like the world is literally broken?

TERENCE: Well, not literally, no. It's more of a metaphor. Imagine for a moment a beautiful mosaic.

KATIE: Okay. I like mosaics. Now imagine that some of the tiles are chipped or broken, maybe even a few missing altogether. The overall picture is still beautiful, but there's a sense of imperfection to it, a feeling that things aren't quite as they should be.

TERENCE: I see what you mean. Like it's still beautiful, but it's got these flaws that kind of stand out.

KATIE: Precisely. And that's sort of how this broken world concept works. It suggests that while we were created for good, for harmony, for this perfect existence, somewhere along the way, things, well, they got a little messed up. And that imperfection, that brokenness, it introduces things like suffering and hardship into the world.

TERENCE: So it's not that God wants us to suffer, but it's more like this side effect of, I don't know, free will, our choices, the fact that we don't always get things right.

KATIE: Exactly. It's like this unavoidable consequence of existing in a world that isn't perfect, A world where free will and choice play a significant role.

TERENCE: Okay, that actually makes a lot of sense. But here's the thing. It doesn't just leave us wallowing in all this brokenness, right? The text then talks about trials as a tool for growth. It's like going through tough times can actually make us stronger, more resilient. Have you ever noticed that?

KATIE: Oh, absolutely. It's a common theme in many spiritual traditions actually.

TERENCE: It's like nobody enjoys going through difficult times, but it's often in those moments that we discover a strength we didn't even know we had. Like we're forced to dig deep and find a way through. And that process, as painful as it can be, can be incredibly transformative.

14

KATIE: The text uses this powerful metaphor of refining precious metals.

TERENCE: Ooh, yes. The refining fire.

KATIE: Exactly. The idea that in order to purify gold to remove its impurities, it has to be subjected to intense heat.

TERENCE: Okay? So we're talking about like really intense heat.

KATIE: It's not a comfortable process, but it's a necessary one to achieve purity.

TERENCE: And it's the same with us in a way.

KATIE: In a way, yes. The text suggests that challenges, while difficult can have a similar refining effect on our character.

TERENCE: It's like we're going into the fire as one version of ourselves kind of rough around the edges, and it's the heat of those trials, those hardships that burns away the impurities leaving behind something stronger and more resilient. Uh, I kind of like that visual, even if it sounds a bit intense.

KATIE: The text even quotes a passage from the book of James reminding us that perseverance through trials produces character. It's in those moments that we often find ourselves relying on our faith on something bigger than ourselves. And that reliance can be incredibly empowering.

15

TERENCE: It's like we discover a well of strength inside of us that we never even knew was there.

KATIE: Exactly.

TERENCE: But here's where things get really interesting for me, Uhhuh

KATIE: <affirmative>,

TERENCE: And maybe a bit paradoxical, the text introduces this idea of free will. We have this incredible gift of choice, right? But then those choices are choices.

KATIE: Mm-Hmm. <affirmative>

TERENCE: Can sometimes be the very things that lead to suffering,

KATIE: Right? Both for ourselves and others.

TERENCE: And that's a tough one to wrap your head around, isn't it? Like we have this freedom to choose, which is amazing, but then those choices have consequences, and sometimes those consequences involve pain, hardship, or even causing suffering for other people. That's a lot of responsibility to carry. It

KATIE: Is, and it's something that the text doesn't shy away from. It acknowledges that tension between God's presence and our very human capacity for both good and bad choices.

TERENCE: Okay, so how do we make sense of that?

KATIE: That's a question we'll continue to explore.

TERENCE: It's like we're not just talking about our own personal struggles here, but the ripple effects of our choices. You know, like one decision can sometimes have these huge unintended consequences that impact other people. It's a lot to consider.

KATIE: It is, and it speaks to the interconnectedness of our lives, how our actions can impact others in ways we might not even realize. But even within that framework, the text doesn't leave us without hope. It emphasizes the unwavering presence of God, even amidst the repercussions of our actions.

TERENCE: Okay? So even when we mess up, even when things get really messy because of choices we made, there's still that sense of what grace, forgiveness.

KATIE: I think those are both beautiful ways to describe it. The text even highlights a passage from Psalm 34.18, which says, the Lord is close to the broken hearted. He rescues those who are crushed in spirit. It's a reminder that even when we feel lost or broken, we're not alone.

TERENCE: It's like no matter how far we stray, no matter how badly we mess up that presence, that love, it's still there. It's a pretty powerful message when you really think about it.

KATIE: It is. It speaks to a love that transcends our human understanding. A love that isn't conditional on our behavior or our ability to get things right all the time. It simply is.

TERENCE: Which brings us to, I think, one of the most challenging parts of the whole. Why do bad things happen to good people? Dilemma the story of Job.

KATIE: Uh, yes, job. His story is a classic for a reason.

TERENCE: It's like if we're supposed to learn from our struggles to grow through hardship, then what about those times when suffering feels completely random?

KATIE: I see your point. It can feel especially difficult to reconcile those kinds of experiences with the idea that everything happens for a reason.

TERENCE: Like Job was by all accounts, a good dude, right? He followed the rules, lived a righteous life, and still got hit with unimaginable suffering, loss, illness, betrayal, you name it. He went through it. It's enough to make anyone question well, everything.

KATIE: And that's precisely the point of job's story. It tackles those very questions head on. It grapples with the mystery of suffering, especially when it feels undeserved or unexplainable.

TERENCE: So what's the answer? Why does this happen even to people who seem to be doing everything right?

KATIE: Well, that's the thing about joke story. It doesn't offer a neat and tidy answer. And in a way that's part of what makes it so powerful. It reflects the reality that sometimes we don't get a clear explanation for our suffering. There are limits to human understanding, especially when it comes to the complexities of the divine plan.

TERENCE: So what are we supposed to do with that? Just to accept that sometimes bad things happen for no reason,

KATIE: Not necessarily for no reason. The text suggests that job's story is less about providing concrete answers and more about encouraging us to shift our perspective.

TERENCE: Okay, so how do we do that? How do we even begin to shift our perspective when we're in the middle of some really tough stuff?

KATIE: It's about moving from a place of needing to know why to a place of trust, trusting that even when we don't understand, even when it feels unfair or overwhelming, there's a bigger picture at play.

TERENCE: So it's more about faith than finding the perfect explanation

KATIE: In a way. Yes, it's about surrendering to the unknown, acknowledging that our human perspective is limited and that there might be a grander narrative unfolding that we can't fully grasp from our current vantage point.

TERENCE: Kind of like those optical illusions where you only see one image until you shift your perspective and then suddenly, boom, there's a whole other picture hidden in plain sight. Maybe we're so focused on the pain, the confusion, the whiny of it all, that we miss the bigger picture, the potential for growth, the possibility that even in the midst of suffering, there's a deeper meaning unfolding.

KATIE: That's a beautiful way to put it. It's not about minimizing the very real pain of suffering, but about expanding our understanding of it. Recognizing that even in those dark and difficult moments, there's still potential for growth, for transformation, and ultimately for hope.

TERENCE: Okay? So even when we're going through something awful, when we're in the thick of it and can't see a way out, there's still this bigger picture of hope.

KATIE: That's what the text seems to suggest.

TERENCE: Um, I'll be honest, sometimes that's hard to see when you're in the middle of a really tough situation.

KATIE: It's a very human response, and the text acknowledges that. It's not about denying the reality of our present suffering, but rather it's inviting us to embrace a wider perspective. It reminds us that our current struggles, however, real and painful, don't define the entirety of our story.

TERENCE: But so yeah, like you were saying earlier, it's just a chapter, not the whole book, even if it feels like an especially long chapter.

KATIE: Exactly. And like any good story, there are peaks and valleys, moments of joy and sorrow, triumph and defeat. But the text assures us that there's a resolution, a sense of restoration and wholeness that awaits us. It even quotes Romans 8.18, which says, I consider that our present sufferings are not worth comparing with the glory that will be revealed in us.

TERENCE: Wow. Okay. That's a powerful image.

KATIE: It is, isn't it?

TERENCE: It's like saying that whatever we're going through now, no matter how big or scary it feels, it's nothing compared to the good stuff that's coming.

KATIE: That's a beautiful way to put it.

TERENCE: So we go into the fire, right? Like we were talking about earlier, as these kind of rough, imperfect beings. We go through these trials, these hard times, and yeah, it's painful. It feels like that intense heat, but it's in that fire that we're refined, we're purified, and we come out stronger, more resilient, and ultimately, that process leads to something truly amazing, something glorious.

KATIE: That's a beautiful way to tie it all together.

TERENCE: So as we wrap up this deep dive, what are some key takeaways we can hold onto? Because honestly, this topic, it's a lot to process.

KATIE: Well, I think the text reminds us that suffering, while universal doesn't have to be meaningless, it invites us to see those tough experiences, those why me, moments through a different lens, to find purpose and even growth in the midst of pain. To trust that even when we don't understand, even when it feels unfair or overwhelming, there's a bigger picture at play. And to remember that even in those dark moments, that hope, that promise of something more is a constant companion,

TERENCE: And that even though it might be really hard sometimes, we can choose how we respond to challenges. We can lean into our faith and we can trust in a plan that's bigger than us.

KATIE: Beautifully said.

TERENCE: Well, on that note, we'll leave you to ponder these profound ideas. And remember, you're not alone in asking those why questions. Keep exploring, keep the conversations going. And until next time, keep diving deep.

THE STUDY GUIDE

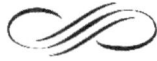

Understanding Suffering: A Biblical Perspective

I. Key Concepts:

The Problem of Suffering: The theological and philosophical challenge of reconciling the existence of a loving, all-powerful God with the reality of pain and suffering in the world.

Free Will: The capacity for humans to make independent choices, even if those choices lead to negative consequences.

Spiritual Growth: The process of developing a deeper relationship with God and becoming more Christ-like, often through trials and challenges.

God's Sovereignty: The belief that God is in ultimate control of the universe and its events, even if we don't always understand His purposes.

Theodicy: An attempt to defend God's goodness and justice in the face of evil and suffering.

II. Short Answer Quiz:

1. Why does the excerpt say that suffering is a part of the human experience?

2. How does the excerpt compare spiritual growth to refining precious metals?

3.   According to the excerpt, how does the concept of free will relate to suffering?

4.   What is the significance of Psalm 34:18 in the context of suffering?

5.   Why is the story of Job significant in discussing the problem of suffering?

6.   How does God respond to Job's questioning of his suffering?

7.   What does Romans 8:18 offer to those struggling with suffering?

8.   What is one way the excerpt suggests that suffering can be a tool for growth?

9.   How does the excerpt describe God's nature in the face of human suffering?

10. According to the excerpt, what is the ultimate hope for those who trust in God?

III. Essay Questions:

1.   Analyze the excerpt's explanation of how free will contributes to suffering. Do you find this argument convincing? Why or why not?

2.   The excerpt draws a parallel between suffering and the refining of precious metals. Discuss the strengths and limitations of this analogy.

3.   Critically examine the excerpt's claim that suffering can be a tool for spiritual growth. Provide examples from your own life or observations to support your points.

4. The excerpt acknowledges that some suffering appears unjust. How can we reconcile the idea of a just and loving God with the existence of seemingly meaningless suffering?

5. Discuss the role of hope in the excerpt's approach to the problem of suffering. How does the promise of future restoration impact our understanding of present pain?

IV. Glossary of Key Terms:

Broken World: A theological concept referring to the state of the world as being marred by sin, suffering, and imperfection.

Comfort: The act of providing solace, encouragement, and support in times of distress or sorrow.

Resilient: The ability to bounce back from adversity, challenges, or setbacks.

Sovereign: Possessing supreme power and authority; ruling over all.

Restoration: The act of returning something to its former, good state; making things right again.

V. Quiz Answer Key

1A. The excerpt emphasizes that suffering is an inherent part of the human experience in a broken world, as acknowledged even by Jesus.

2A. The excerpt uses the analogy of refining precious metals to illustrate how trials and difficulties can test and purify our faith, leading to spiritual growth.

3A. Free will, according to the excerpt, means humans can make choices that lead to suffering, both for themselves and others.

4A. Psalm 34:18 emphasizes that God is not indifferent to suffering but is close to the brokenhearted and offers comfort.

5A. Job's story highlights the theological problem of undeserved suffering, as he was righteous yet faced immense hardship.

6A. God responds to Job by emphasizing His sovereign power and wisdom, reminding Job that His ways are beyond human comprehension.

7A. Romans 8:18 provides hope by emphasizing that future joy in Christ will outweigh present suffering.

8A. Suffering, as the excerpt suggests, can lead to growth by revealing our dependence on God and building resilience.

9A. The excerpt portrays God as being near to those who suffer, offering comfort, hope, and ultimately, restoration.

10A. The excerpt underscores that those who trust God have the hope of a future where suffering is no more and all wrongs are made right.

FREQUENTLY ASKED QUESTIONS

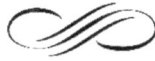

1. Why do bad things happen if God is good?

This is a question humans have grappled with for centuries. Suffering is a part of life in a broken world, and its presence doesn't mean God is absent or uncaring. The Bible reminds us that we will face hardship in this life (John 16:33), but God is always with us through it.

2. Can suffering have a purpose?

Yes, the Bible suggests that suffering can be a catalyst for growth and refinement of our faith (James 1:2-3). Just as refining precious metals involves intense heat, trials can reveal our true selves and push us to rely more on God, making us stronger and more resilient.

3. How does free will factor into suffering?

God granted humanity free will, and with that comes the possibility of making choices that lead to suffering, both for ourselves and others. While this doesn't mean God is indifferent to pain, it acknowledges the complexities of a world where individuals make choices with varying consequences.

4. What about when suffering seems entirely unjust?

The book of Job addresses this directly. Job, a righteous man, endured immense suffering, showing that sometimes pain is not a direct result of our actions. While we may not always understand the reasons, God is still present and cares for us deeply.

5. Is God moved by our suffering?

Yes, the Bible emphasizes God's compassion for those who suffer. Psalm 34:18 assures us that "The Lord is close to the brokenhearted; he rescues those whose spirits are crushed." His love and comfort are constant sources of strength during difficult times.

6. What can we learn from Job's response to suffering?

Job's story highlights the importance of trusting God's sovereignty, even when we don't understand His plans. Despite his pain, Job chose to trust in God's wisdom and power, ultimately finding peace in surrender and faith.

7. Does suffering have an end?

For those who believe, suffering is not the end. Romans 8:18 offers hope for a future where God will make all things right, a time of restoration and joy that surpasses any earthly pain. This promise doesn't diminish present suffering but offers an eternal perspective.

8. What is the key takeaway when facing hardship?

While the question of suffering is complex, remember that God is present, compassionate, and sovereign. Trust in His plan, even when it's unclear. Lean on His promises of growth through trials and the ultimate hope of a future free from pain.

CHAPTER TWO

BELIEF #2

How does God use the problems and struggles in my life for His ultimate good and mine?

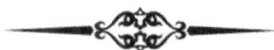

———— ◆ ————

CHAPTER TWO / BELIEF #2 – TABLE OF CONTENTS

BELIEF #2

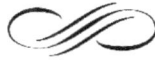

How does God use the problems and struggles in my life for His ultimate good and mine?

Life is full of challenges, difficulties, and unexpected twists. At times, it can feel overwhelming and leave us wondering, "Why is this happening to me?" However, the Bible teaches us that **God is not absent in our struggles**. In fact, He often uses these very difficulties to bring about something greater—both for His purposes and for our own personal growth.

One of the most comforting truths in the Bible is that **God has a plan for each of our lives,** and nothing that happens is outside of His control. The Apostle Paul reminds us of this in Romans 8:28 (The Message): "That's why we can be so sure that every detail in our lives of love for God is worked into something good." This verse doesn't suggest that everything in life will be easy or pain-free. Instead, it assures us that **God can take even the most difficult circumstances and use them for our ultimate good.**

It's important to understand that God's definition of "good" might not always align with our own. While we might long for comfort, ease, or success, God is more concerned with our character, our faith, and our relationship with Him. Struggles often become the very tools He uses to refine these aspects of our lives.

31

Consider the story of Joseph in the Old Testament. Joseph faced betrayal by his brothers, slavery, false accusations, and imprisonment. At any point, he could have given in to despair, wondering how any good could come from such hardship. But later in his life, when Joseph was in a position of power and his brothers feared retribution, he told them in Genesis 50:20 (The Message), "Don't you see, you planned evil against me but God used those same plans for my good, as you see all around you right now—life for many people." Joseph recognized that **God had a bigger picture in mind, one that went beyond his personal pain and suffering.**

God also uses struggles to draw us closer to Him. When life is going smoothly, it's easy to become self-reliant or complacent. But when we face challenges, we often turn to God in prayer, seeking His help, guidance, and comfort. The Psalmist writes in Psalm 46:1 (The Message), "God is a safe place to hide, ready to help when we need him." Difficult times remind us of our need for God and can <u>deepen our relationship with Him</u> as we learn to trust Him more fully.

Moreover, <u>struggles can build our faith</u>. James 1:2-4 (The Message) says, "Consider it a sheer gift, friends, when tests and challenges come at you from all sides. You know that under pressure, your faith-life is forced into the open and shows its true colors. So don't try to get out of anything prematurely. Let it do its work so you become mature and well-developed, not deficient in any way." **James is not suggesting that we enjoy suffering, but rather that we see it as an opportunity for growth.** Through these experiences, our faith is strengthened, and we become more resilient.

Finally, **the struggles we endure can also equip us to help others.** When we have walked through the valley of hardship and come out on the other side, we are in a unique position to offer comfort and encouragement to those facing similar trials. Paul speaks to this in 2 Corinthians 1:3-4 (The Message): "All praise to the God and Father of our Master, Jesus the Messiah! Father of all mercy! God of all healing counsel! He comes alongside us when we go through hard times, and before you know it, he brings us alongside someone else who is going through hard times so that we can be there for that person just as God was there for us."

While we may not always understand why we face certain struggles in life, we can be confident that God is using them for a greater purpose. He is shaping us, strengthening our faith, drawing us closer to Him, and preparing us to help others. **As we trust in His plan, we can rest in the assurance that He is working all things together for our ultimate good.** Even in the midst of trials, we are never alone, and our struggles are never wasted in the hands of a loving and sovereign God.

THE PODCAST TRANSCRIPT

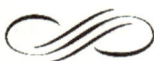

KATIE: Ever feel like you're stuck in one of those spinning carnival rides? You know, the, the ones that just won't quit life can feel like that sometimes. Right? Full of those unexpected twists and turns. But what if, and stay with me here. What if the, those curve balls, those struggles, those moments that make you wanna scream? What if they're actually part of something bigger?

TERENCE: Hmm. I like where you're going with this.

KATIE: Well, today we're diving deep into a text that explores how a biblical perspective views those inevitable bumps in the road and how God might be using them, using all of it for good.

TERENCE: Okay, now you've got my attention.

KATIE: So this source, it really digs into the idea that even when things seem messy, there's a plan.

TERENCE: Right? Right.

KATIE: And not just any plan, but God's plan.

TERENCE: Yeah. But, and here's the thing.

KATIE: Yeah.

TERENCE: His plan and our plan

KATIE: Totally different. Right.

TERENCE: Often miles apart, you see, we usually think good equals comfortable, successful, you know, smooth sailing. But God's view it's way bigger.

KATIE: Way bigger.

TERENCE: He's playing the long game. Yeah. He's focused on our character, our spiritual growth, our relationship with him, and honestly, sometimes the path to get there. Mm-Hmm. <affirmative>. It's not always pretty.

KATIE: Definitely not always Instagram worthy, that's for sure. Mm-Hmm. <affirmative>. It makes sense when you explain it like that, but it's still tough to swallow when you're in the middle of a struggle, it's easy to fall into that trap of, if God has a plan, why does it involve so much pain?

TERENCE: Oh, 100%. It's human nature, right?

KATIE: Yeah.

TERENCE: We want control, we want answers. Yeah. Why me? Why Now we've all been there, but think about it, some of the most pivotal moments of growth for people, for communities, for entire nations, even those moments often came after intense

KATIE: Challenges. It's like that verse, Romans 8.28, and we know that in all things, God works for the good of those who love him, who have been called according to his purpose. It gets quoted a lot that verse, but I think it's easy to miss the nuance there.

TERENCE: Absolutely. There's a lot packed in there.

KATIE: It doesn't say, we won't face difficulties, does it?

TERENCE: Nope. It doesn't. It's not saying, Hey, no hardship for you, you're good. It's about God's ability to take those tough moments, the messy ones. Mm-hmm. Even the painful ones. And make the meaningful, it's like imagine a master tapestry, weaver. We might just see a jumbled mess of threads, but they see the potential for this intricate beautiful design.

KATIE: So it's less about avoiding the tough stuff and more about trusting that God can use it for good, even when we can't see the whole picture yet.

TERENCE: Exactly.

KATIE: Okay. I'm starting to see it.

TERENCE: And speaking of trusting in God's plan, even when it's hard, have you ever thought about Joseph in the Old Testament?

KATIE: Oh, are you kidding? Talk about a life of ups and downs, betrayed by his brothers sold into slavery, falsely accused. His story's like, it's like something you'd see in a movie.

TERENCE: Right? Imagine going through even one of those things. But Joseph, he went through all

36

of it. He faced each challenge one after another. But here's the thing, he never became bitter. He never lost hope. He held onto his faith and those trials, as often as they were, they ended up the catalyst for something incredible.

KATIE: Right. He ends up in a position of power in Egypt and saves countless lives, including his families during a famine. It's kind of mind blowing to think those struggles, as awful as they were, their struggles were part of a much bigger plan, A plan that ultimately brought about so much good. It reminds me of that saying, we admire the beauty of a butterfly, but we forget about the transformation it took to get there. Joseph's story is like that, right? This powerful reminder that some of the most beautiful outcomes come from going through some dark times.

TERENCE: Exactly. And it wasn't just about the big picture stuff like saving a nation. Think about Joseph's own personal journey.

KATIE: Oh yeah, good point.

TERENCE: He learned resilience, he learned forgiveness.

KATIE: Yeah.

TERENCE: And his trust in God unwavering, even when he couldn't see what was coming next.

KATIE: It's easy to say that now, but But to actually live it, that's another thing altogether,

TERENCE: Right? You have to dig deep, find that inner strength when things get rough.

KATIE: Yeah.

TERENCE: We've all been there.

KATIE: Absolutely. It's like that verse, Psalm 46.1, God is our refuge and strength and ever present help and trouble. There's something so comforting about that image knowing that no matter what's going on, God is our safe place. But you know what? Sometimes it takes those storms, those challenges to make us actually seek out that refuge, don't you think?

TERENCE: Totally. It's easy to feel self-sufficient when life is good. Yeah. You know, when things are smooth sailing, but those desperate moments, Hmm. The ones that strip us bare and make us realize how little control we really have. Those are often the moments when we truly understand how much we need God, the

KATIE: Humbling

TERENCE: We let go, we surrender that need to be in control, and suddenly we're open to depending on something bigger than ourselves, and you know what happens then? Our faith, it's refined, made stronger, tested by fire. It's

KATIE: Like James says, right in his letter, he actually says it's pure joy to go through trials and challenges. Now, I gotta be honest with you, joy isn't exactly the first thing I think of when I'm struggling

TERENCE: <laugh>, right? It doesn't exactly scream party time, but if you look at what James is saying in James 1.2 to four, he's not celebrating suffering. He's talking about the power of perseverance. He's like, listen, he challenges are part of life, but instead of letting them crush you, what if you saw them as a chance to grow, to build character, to strengthen your resilience and deepen your trust in God?

KATIE: Okay. Yeah. It's a total perspective shift. It's not about pretending things are fine when they're not. It's about choosing to see the potential for growth right in the middle of it.

TERENCE: Yes. And there's another really beautiful aspect to this whole idea of God using struggles for good, and it goes beyond just our own personal growth. It's about how these very experiences can equip us to help other people who are going through similar things.

KATIE: Oh man, I've so been there a few years ago. I went through a really hard time and so many people reached out sharing their stories about how they overcame similar situations. Just knowing I wasn't alone was huge, and it made me wanna do the same for others. You know, be that person for someone else.

TERENCE: It's this beautiful ripple effect, and it's something Paul wrote about too in two Corinthians 1.3 to four. He says, praise be to the God and father of our Lord Jesus Christ, the father of compassion and the God of all comfort, who comforts us in all our troubles so that we can comfort those in any trouble with the comfort we ourselves receive from God.

KATIE: Wow. That's powerful. It's like our experiences, even the painful ones, become this source of comfort and understanding that we can then share. We say, Hey, I've been there. I get it. You're not alone. And that connection, that empathy, that's powerful stuff.

TERENCE: Absolutely. It's the golden rule in action, right? Love your neighbor as yourself. Weep with those who weep. Offer a helping hand, not just from a place of knowing, but from a place of understanding. And you only get that kind of understanding by going through the fire yourself.

KATIE: It's like those stars we get, you know, like battle wounds, but from facing tough times, they become these badges of honor in a way, right. Reminders of what we survived and how much stronger we became because of it.

TERENCE: Right. They show what we've overcome and they can be these bridges to other people who are going through similar things.

KATIE: Totally. There's this quote, I love it. It says, the wound is the place where the light enters you. And it's true, right? It's often those broken

40

places, the places where we had to face pain and uncertainty. That's where we find out who we really are, what our faith is really made of.

TERENCE: Yeah. And those experiences can make us incredibly strong and resilient too. Think about it, when you've gone through something hard and come out on the other side, you know you can handle anything. You've got this inner strength, this confidence that can't be shaken by every little thing.

KATIE: So as tempting as it is to want to avoid difficult times altogether, to just pray for smooth sailing all the time, maybe there's something to embracing those challenges, seeing them as opportunities to grow, connect with others, find our purpose.

TERENCE: Absolutely. It's a perspective shift. You know, instead of asking, why me when something bad happens, what if we ask, what is God trying to teach me here? How could this actually be part of his plan to shape me, to mold me into who I'm supposed to be?

KATIE: That is a powerful question. Instead of focusing on how much it hurts, we can look for how we can grow from it. Trusting that even when we don't understand, God is still in control. He still has a plan.

TERENCE: We have to let go of trying to understand everything, you know, embrace the mystery of it all, and trust that even if things seem

41

messy right now, God can take those pieces, those broken pieces, and make them into something beautiful and purposeful.

KATIE: It's like we're all part of this huge tapestry, and even those threads that seem dark or out of place, they still have a part to play in the overall picture. So to everyone listening, if you're carrying some of those heavier threads right now, the ones that weigh you down and make you unsure, just remember this. You're not alone

TERENCE: In those very struggles. Those times of hardship and uncertainty, they can actually refine you, they can make you stronger, and they can bring you closer to God in ways you never imagined possible.

KATIE: They might even be preparing you to offer hope and encouragement to someone else going through something similar. So don't give up even when it hurts. Remember, God is still working everything together for good.

TERENCE: Absolutely. And with that, here's something to think about. What if the things you see as setbacks are actually set ups setups for God to do his greatest work in and through you.

KATIE: Thanks for joining us today for this deep dive, everyone.

THE STUDY GUIDE

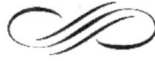

God's Purpose in Our Struggles: A Study Guide

I. Quiz

1. According to Romans 8:28, what does God work into something good?

2. How does God's definition of "good" differ from our own?

3. What is significant about Joseph's statement to his brothers in Genesis 50:20?

4. How can difficult times actually strengthen our relationship with God?

5. Explain the analogy used in James 1:2-4 to describe the effect of trials on our faith.

6. How does the experience of overcoming hardship equip us to help others?

7. What is the main idea presented in 2 Corinthians 1:3-4?

8. Why might we not always understand the reasons behind our struggles?

9. What assurance can we find despite not fully understanding our circumstances?

10. What is the ultimate message of hope offered in this excerpt?

II. Answer Key

1A. Romans 8:28 assures us that God works every detail in our lives of love for Him into something good.

2A. While we often equate "good" with comfort and ease, God prioritizes the development of our character, faith, and relationship with Him.

3A. Joseph acknowledges that while his brothers intended to harm him, God used their actions for a greater good, saving lives and fulfilling His purpose.

4A. Challenges often drive us to seek God's help, guidance, and comfort through prayer, deepening our dependence on Him and strengthening our relationship.

5A. James compares trials to pressure that reveals the true nature of our faith, refining and strengthening it like metal tested in fire.

6A. Going through hardships gives us empathy and allows us to offer genuine comfort, encouragement, and guidance to those facing similar situations.

7A. This passage highlights God's compassion in comforting us during trials so that we, in turn, can comfort others, demonstrating a ripple effect of His grace.

8A. Our limited human perspective often prevents us from grasping God's greater plan and the reasons behind our struggles.

9A. Despite not always understanding, we can find assurance in knowing that God is in control, working all things together for our good as we trust in Him.

10A. Even in the midst of hardship, we are never alone; God is present, our struggles are not wasted, and He is working to bring about His ultimate good in our lives.

III. Essay Questions

1. Analyze the biblical example of Joseph. How does his story illustrate God's ability to transform suffering into something good?

2. Discuss the relationship between struggles, faith, and personal growth. How do trials refine these aspects of our lives according to the excerpt?

3. Explain the concept of God's "good" differing from our own understanding. How can we reconcile our desire for ease with God's desire for our spiritual development?

4. Explore the idea that our struggles can be used to help others. How does this perspective provide comfort and purpose in the midst of hardship?

5. Reflect on a personal experience where you believe God used a difficult situation for a greater good. How did this experience impact your faith and understanding of God's character?

IV. Glossary of Key Terms

Sovereign: Possessing supreme power and authority.

Refine: To improve something by removing its flaws or impurities.

Resilient: Able to withstand or recover quickly from difficult conditions.

Complacent: Showing smug or uncritical satisfaction with oneself.

Retribution: Punishment inflicted on someone as vengeance for a wrong or criminal act.

Equip: To provide someone with the necessary skills or abilities.

Assurance: A positive declaration intended to give confidence.

FREQUENTLY ASKED QUESTIONS

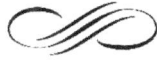

1. Why does life feel so difficult sometimes?

Life is inherently filled with challenges, disappointments, and unexpected events. While these experiences can be painful and leave us questioning their purpose, the Bible teaches that God is present even in our darkest moments. He uses these trials to shape us, strengthen our faith, and draw us closer to Him.

2. Does God really have a plan for my life, even when things are difficult?

Yes, the Bible assures us that God has a plan for each of us, and nothing falls outside His control. Romans 8:28 states that God works all things together for good for those who love Him. This doesn't mean life will be easy, but it does mean that He can use even the most challenging circumstances for our ultimate benefit.

3. What does God consider "good" in the midst of my struggles?

God's definition of "good" might differ from ours. While we often desire comfort and ease, God prioritizes our spiritual growth, character development, and deepening relationship with Him. Our struggles can become the very tools He uses to refine these essential aspects of our lives.

4. How can I trust God's plan when I don't understand what's happening?

The story of Joseph in the Old Testament provides a powerful example. He endured betrayal, slavery, and imprisonment. Yet, he ultimately recognized God's hand in orchestrating events for a greater purpose. Like Joseph, we can trust that God's plans are for our good, even when we lack complete understanding.

5. How can struggles actually bring me closer to God?

When life is smooth sailing, it's easy to become self-reliant and forget our need for God. However, challenges often drive us to seek Him through prayer, dependence, and a desire for His comfort. This dependence deepens our relationship with Him as we learn to trust Him more fully.

6. What does it mean that my faith is tested through hardship?

James 1:2-4 encourages us to view trials as opportunities for spiritual growth. Just as pressure reveals the true strength of a material, challenges reveal and refine the authenticity of our faith. We emerge from these experiences stronger, more resilient, and more deeply rooted in our trust in God.

7. Can my struggles actually benefit others?

Yes, our personal experiences with hardship equip us to empathize with and support others facing similar challenges. 2 Corinthians 1:3-4 emphasizes that God comforts us in our trials so that we, in turn, can comfort others with the same comfort we received. Our struggles become testimonies of God's faithfulness and sources of encouragement for those around us.

8. What can I hold onto when I feel overwhelmed by life's difficulties?

Remember that even in the midst of trials, you are not alone. God is present, working all things together for your good. He uses your struggles to draw you closer to Him, strengthen your faith, and equip you to help others. Embrace His promise that He will never leave or forsake you, and trust that He is using every experience to shape you into the person He created you to be.

CHAPTER THREE

BELIEF #3

Why God always loves you unconditionally?

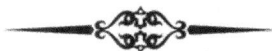

———— ❧❦❧ ————

CHAPTER THREE / BELIEF #3 – TABLE OF CONTENTS

BELIEF #3

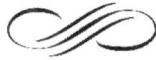

Why God always loves you unconditionally?

In our daily lives, we often find ourselves trying to earn love and acceptance. Whether it's through our actions, words, or achievements, there's a constant pressure to prove that we are worthy of love. But when it comes to God's love, the Bible teaches us something radically different. God's love is not something we have to earn; it is freely given. This is the incredible truth of unconditional love—God always loves you, no matter what.

God's Love is Unchanging

One of the most remarkable aspects of God's love is that it is constant. Human love can be fickle, changing with circumstances, moods, or misunderstandings. But God's love is not like that. It is unchanging and everlasting. The Bible says in Jeremiah 31:3 (The Message), "God told them, 'I've never quit loving you and never will. Expect love, love, and more love!'" This verse reveals the depth and permanence of God's love. He doesn't love us because of who we are or what we've done; He loves us because of who He is. His love is an unbreakable promise, grounded in His unchanging nature.

God's Love is Unconditional

Another key aspect of God's love is that it is unconditional. This means that there are no conditions or prerequisites for God to love us. He doesn't wait for us to

53

get our lives in order, to stop sinning, or to prove our worth before He extends His love to us. Romans 5:8 (The Message) reminds us, "But God put His love on the line for us by offering His Son in sacrificial death while we were of no use whatever to Him." Even when we were far from Him, lost in our sins, God loved us enough to send His Son to die for us. This shows that His love is not based on our performance or righteousness; it is a gift that He gives freely.

God's Love is Personal

God's love is also deeply personal. He knows each of us intimately—our fears, our failures, our hopes, and our dreams—and He loves us just the same. The Bible tells us in Psalm 139:1-3 (The Message), "God, investigate my life; get all the facts firsthand. I'm an open book to you; even from a distance, you know what I'm thinking. You know when I leave and when I get back; I'm never out of your sight." God's love is not distant or generic; it is specific and personal. He knows us better than we know ourselves, and yet His love for us never wavers. He sees our flaws and our shortcomings, but He also sees our potential and the person He created us to be. His love is a constant presence in our lives, guiding, protecting, and comforting us.

God's Love Transforms Us

Understanding God's unconditional love can have a profound impact on our lives. When we realize that we are loved by God just as we are, it frees us from the need to perform or earn His approval. We don't have to be perfect to be loved by God. His love gives us the confidence to face our fears and challenges, knowing that we are never alone. This love also motivates us to love others in the same way. As we experience God's unconditional love, we are inspired to extend that love to those around us, creating a ripple effect of love and grace.

Conclusion

God's love for you is a foundational truth that can transform your life. It is unchanging, unconditional, and deeply personal. The Bible assures us that no matter where we are in life or what we have done, God's love is always with us. Jeremiah 31:3, Romans 5:8, and Psalm 139:1-3 remind us of this incredible truth: God's love is not something we earn; it is a gift that He freely gives because of who He is. Embracing this love can change the way we see ourselves, our circumstances, and the world around us. So, rest in the knowledge that you are always loved by God—unconditionally, endlessly, and completely.

THE PODCAST TRANSCRIPT

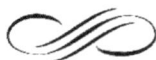

TERENCE: Alright, so today we're gonna do a deep dive on something, you know, we hear about all the time, God's unconditional love. But we're gonna use this, uh, this excerpt, right? It's called B-I-F-B-C-C Stack three, and really try to like go a little deeper with it. Yeah.

KATIE: B-I-F-B-C-C stack Three. I'll admit that title leaves me with more questions than answers, but the concept itself, God's unconditional love, that's something I'm always ready to explore.

TERENCE: Absolutely. Me too. And this, this excerpt it, uh, it starts out, it talks about this thing we probably all feel this pressure to like, prove we deserve love, you

KATIE: Know? Yeah. Like,

TERENCE: We gotta earn it, measure up somehow.

KATIE: Yeah, for sure.

TERENCE: And for me, that's, that's definitely something I've struggled with.

KATIE: Well, it makes sense though, right? If you think about it like, way back when with our early ancestors belonging to a group, to a tribe, it wasn't just about like fitting in, it was about survival.

TERENCE: Oh, totally.

KATIE: So this deep need for approval that we all have, it's, it's practically woven into our DNA.

TERENCE: Wow. That's, that's a really interesting way to look at it.

KATIE: Yeah.

TERENCE: But, but I guess the problem comes in when, when that instinct that need to be loved starts to like, make us believe that love is something we have to earn.

KATIE: Exactly. And that's where things can get messy.

TERENCE: It's like this constant pressure, this feeling of I'll be loved, IF

KATIE: Right. And that's, I think where this idea of God's love, at least how this excerpt talks about it, it's like completely different.

TERENCE: Yeah. It's like, it totally flips the script on how we usually think about love. Right.

KATIE: Absolutely. This excerpt, it really hones in on three big things about God's love. It's unchanging, it's unconditional and it's personal. So should we, uh, should we take a closer look at each of those?

TERENCE: Yeah. Let's do it. So unchanging. What makes God's love different from like, the love we experience with other people?

KATIE: Well, human love is powerful, don't get me wrong, but it's also, how do I say this? It's kind of fickle sometimes, right? You know, things change. People change and sometimes that means the love changes too.

TERENCE: So you're saying that like God's love doesn't depend on any of that.

KATIE: Exactly. It doesn't matter what we do. God's love for us according to this, it stays the same.

TERENCE: Okay. So even when we mess up, make bad choices, God still loves us the same. That's, that's kind of hard to wrap my head around.

KATIE: It is this excerpt, it uses a verse from Jeremiah chapter 31 verse three. It says, I have loved you with an everlasting love, therefore I have continued my faithfulness to you.

TERENCE: Wow. That's, that's powerful. Okay. So that's unchanging. Now unconditional love. This one almost feels too good to be true. Like really no strings attached.

KATIE: Right. It sounds kind of crazy, but that's what this excerpt is saying. It's like, there's absolutely nothing you have to do to earn God's love. He just loves you.

TERENCE: So like, no matter what I do, no matter what I believe, it doesn't matter.

KATIE: It really doesn't. The excerpt uses this really powerful image from Romans 5.8. It says, God shows his love for us in that while we were still sinners, Christ died for us.

TERENCE: So even before we had a chance to like, get things right, to prove anything, it was already there.

KATIE: Already there. Yeah. That's unconditional love my friend. It's not a reward, it's just who God is.

TERENCE: That's amazing. I mean, think about it. We don't have to do anything to earn it.

KATIE: It's pretty mind blowing. Right. And uh, speaking of mind blowing, that actually brings us to the third thing this excerpt talks about. It's that God's love. It's not just this like general, you know, love for humanity thing,

TERENCE: Right.

KATIE: It's personal. Like he knows us each individually and loves us that way.

TERENCE: So it's not like we all just get the same, I know. Like a standard serving of love and that's it.

KATIE: No, not at all. And this excerpt, it uses this example from psalms, Psalm 1 39 verse one through three. It talks about how God knows us completely inside and out, our thoughts, what we do. Everything

TERENCE: That's kind of intense when you really think about it.

KATIE: It is. It's like he sees us even better than we see ourselves. And uh, and here's the amazing part. Yeah. Even knowing everything about us, all our flaws and everything, he still loves us completely.

TERENCE: Wow. So that means that we can be totally ourselves, quirks and all, and God's love for us. It doesn't change. But how do we even start to like live that out? I mean, knowing this should change how we live, shouldn't it?

KATIE: You would think so, right? That's the real question here, I think. And thankfully this excerpt, it doesn't just leave us hanging with these big ideas.

TERENCE: That's he good.

KATIE: Yeah. It actually gets really practical and says that really getting this, this truth about God's unconditional love, it can be incredibly freeing.

TERENCE: Freeing how? In what ways? Okay.

KATIE: So imagine this, all that pressure we feel to perform, to earn love by like doing all the right things or being perfect, it just disappears.

TERENCE: Wow. I like the sound of that,

KATIE: Right?

TERENCE: Yeah.

KATIE: Because we realize that we're already loved completely just as we are right now. So we can finally relax and just, just be ourselves.

TERENCE: Right? Yeah. That would be amazing. I could see how that would be so freeing to not feel like we have to earn God's love.

KATIE: It's a game changer. And it doesn't stop there. This freedom, it impacts everything. Relationships, how we see ourselves, everything.

TERENCE: How so?

KATIE: Well for one, we can be more genuine in our relationships, right? We don't have to pretend or put on a show.

TERENCE: Right. Because we know deep down we're already loved unconditionally. So we don't need that validation from others.

KATIE: Exactly. And then we can go after what we're passionate about without this fear of failing, you know?

TERENCE: Mm-Hmm. <affirmative>.

KATIE: Because our worth, it's not tied to our accomplishments anymore. It's already solid.

TERENCE: Hmm. That's a good point. And I guess it also helps us to accept our imperfections. 'cause we realize that God loves us imperfections and all.

KATIE: Exactly. It's not about pretending to be perfect, but about being fully known and loved for who we truly are. Flaws and all.

TERENCE: So it's not just about feeling good, right? Mm-Hmm. <affirmative>, it's been a totally different way of living and seeing

KATIE: Ourselves. You got it. And get this, this excerpt, it says that when we really experience this kind of love, this unconditional love from God, it inspires us to do the same for others.

TERENCE: Oh wow. That's beautiful. So it's like this ripple effect. We experience it and then we can't help but share it with others.

KATIE: That's it. It's like this amazing cycle. We receive this incredible unconditional love from God and then it overflows from us to the people around us.

TERENCE: It's like we become these like living examples of that love just, just by experiencing it ourselves. You know?

KATIE: I love that. And it really speaks to just how powerful this concept is, right? It's not just some nice idea we can think about. It's, it's something that has the potential to totally change us from the inside out and, and then that change, it impacts the world around us.

TERENCE: Yeah, absolutely. And I think we've done a really good job in this deep dive. Like looking at this idea of God's unconditional love from, from all angles talked about the, the theology behind it, but also how it actually plays out in our lives. Right? You know, it's not just theoretical, it's real. So as we're kind of wrapping things up here, what would you say is the most important thing for our listeners to take away from all of

KATIE: This? That's a great question. We've covered a lot of ground today, but if I had to pick just one thing, it would be this God's love for you. It's constant. It's not based on anything you do or how you feel or even how well you understand it. It just is. And once you really get that, it changes everything. Man.

TERENCE: That is so good. It's like this, this unshakeable always their love that we can always turn to no matter what.

KATIE: Exactly. And realizing that it opens up so much freedom and possibility in our lives.

TERENCE: This deep dive has definitely given me a lot to think about. And I'm sure our listeners feel the same way,

KATIE: Right?

TERENCE: Like if, if God's love really is this unconditional, this unshakeable, how does that change how we treat ourselves, how we face challenges, how we love other people, even when it's tough?

KATIE: Those are great questions. And you know what? I have a feeling the answers to those questions, they'll show up in the most amazing ways as we keep going on this journey of faith and, and keep learning and growing.

TERENCE: That's a great place to end it. So to everyone listening, thank you so much for joining us for this deep dive into God's unconditional love. We hope this conversation has sparked some new thoughts and encouraged you to really, truly embrace that love in your own lives. Until next time, keep exploring, keep asking questions, and keep on loving.

THE STUDY GUIDE

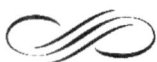

Understanding God's Unconditional Love.

I. Quiz

Instructions: Answer the following questions in 2-3 sentences based on the provided excerpt.

1. How does God's love differ from human love, as described in the text?

2. What makes God's love unchanging, according to the provided verses?

3. Explain the meaning of unconditional love in the context of God's love for humanity.

4. Using Psalm 139:1-3, explain how the text describes God's intimate knowledge of us.

5. How does God's love influence our actions towards others?

6. What is the central message of Jeremiah 31:3?

7. According to Romans 5:8, when did God demonstrate His love for us?

8. Why does God love us, according to the text?

9. How can understanding God's unconditional love transform our lives?

10. What is the key takeaway message the text wants readers to embrace?

II. Answer Key

1A. Unlike human love which can be inconsistent and dependent on circumstances, God's love is described as constant and unwavering, unaffected by our actions.

2A. God's love is unchanging because it is rooted in His own nature. It's not dependent on us, but on who He is, making it a constant and everlasting love.

3A. Unconditional love means God's love is not earned or deserved. There are no conditions or prerequisites for us to receive it; He loves us simply because He chooses to.

4A. These verses highlight God's intimate and personal knowledge of us. He sees our thoughts, actions, and even our whereabouts, emphasizing a deep and personal awareness of our beings.

5A. As we experience God's unconditional love, we are inspired to share that same love with others, fostering a sense of generosity and grace in our interactions.

6A. This verse emphasizes the constant and unwavering nature of God's love, assuring us that He has never stopped loving us and never will, promising "love, love, and more love."

7A. The verse states God demonstrated His love while we were "of no use whatever to Him," highlighting that His love was given freely while we were still sinners, undeserving of His grace.

8A. The text emphasizes that God loves us not because of who we are or what we do, but because of who He is. His love is an inherent aspect of His being, freely given.

9A. Understanding God's unconditional love can liberate us from the pressure of performance or earning His approval. This allows us to live with confidence, knowing we are loved regardless of our flaws.

10A. The text encourages readers to find peace and security in knowing that God's love is unwavering, unconditional, and always accessible, regardless of our life circumstances.

III. Essay Questions

1. Discuss the significance of God's unchanging love in the context of human experiences of love and loss.

2. Analyze the implications of God's unconditional love for our understanding of sin and redemption.

3. Explore how the personal nature of God's love, as described in Psalm 139:1-3, can impact our relationship with Him.

4. How does the text's message of God's unconditional love challenge or affirm your own beliefs about God?

5. In a world often driven by conditional love and acceptance, what are the practical ways we can live out the unconditional love of God in our daily lives?

IV. Glossary of Key Terms

Unconditional Love: Love that is given freely and without any conditions or prerequisites. It is not based on the worthiness of the recipient or their actions.

Everlasting Love: Love that is eternal and never-ending. It is not bound by time or circumstance.

Intimate Knowledge: A deep and personal understanding of someone's thoughts, feelings, and motivations.

Transform: To undergo a complete change in character, nature, or appearance.

Grace: Unmerited favor or kindness. It is a gift from God that we do not deserve.

Redemption: The act of being saved from sin and its consequences. This is made possible through Jesus Christ's sacrifice.

FREQUENTLY ASKED QUESTIONS

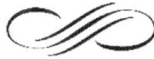

1. Why does God love me unconditionally?

God's love is not dependent on you or your actions. He loves you because it is part of His nature. His love is a free gift, not something you earn.

2. Does God's love ever change?

Unlike human love, God's love is unchanging and everlasting. Jeremiah 31:3 says, "I've never quit loving you and never will. Expect love, love, and more love!" This promise is rooted in His constant and unwavering character.

3. Do I have to do anything to be worthy of God's love?

No, God's love is unconditional. You don't have to be perfect, stop sinning, or prove yourself in any way. Romans 5:8 tells us that God demonstrated His love while we were still sinners, far from deserving it.

4. Does God really know and love me personally?

Yes, God's love is deeply personal. Psalm 139:1-3 reminds us that He knows our thoughts, our comings and goings – He sees every aspect of who we are, and loves us intimately.

5. How can understanding God's unconditional love change my life?

Knowing you are completely loved by God can be incredibly freeing. It releases you from the pressure of striving for approval. You can face challenges with confidence, knowing you are never alone.

6. How does God's love inspire us to love others?

Experiencing God's unconditional love motivates us to extend that same grace and compassion to those around us. It creates a ripple effect, spreading love and acceptance.

7. What are some Bible verses that demonstrate God's unconditional love?

> **Jeremiah 31:3:** "God told them, 'I've never quit loving you and never will. Expect love, love, and more love!'"

> **Romans 5:8:** "But God put His love on the line for us by offering His Son in sacrificial death while we were of no use whatever to Him."

> **Psalm 139:1-3:** "God, investigate my life; get all the facts firsthand. I'm an open book to you; even from a distance, you know what I'm thinking. You know when I leave and when I get back; I'm never out of your sight."

8. How can I fully embrace God's unconditional love?

Spend time reading the Bible and reflecting on scriptures that speak about God's love. Talk to Him in prayer, expressing your gratitude for His unwavering affection. Allow His love to transform your thoughts, actions, and relationships with others.

CHAPTER FOUR

BELIEF #4

The three reasons God is always with you and will never leave you.

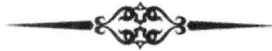

CHAPTER FOUR / BELIEF #4 – TABLE OF CONTENTS

BELIEF #4

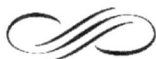

The three reasons God is always with you and will never leave you.

The Bible teaches us that God is always with us and will never leave us, a truth that is both comforting and empowering. Understanding this can bring peace to our hearts and give us the strength to face any challenge. Let's explore three reasons why God is always with us and will never leave us, supported by Scripture.

First, God's presence is a promise. From the beginning of time, God has promised to be with His people. This isn't just a temporary assurance; it's an eternal promise. One powerful reminder of this is found in the book of Joshua. As Joshua was preparing to lead the Israelites into the Promised Land, God spoke directly to him, saying, "I'll be with you. I won't give up on you; I won't leave you" (Joshua 1:5, MSG). This promise wasn't just for Joshua; it's for all of us. God's commitment to His people is unwavering. He doesn't just watch from a distance; He actively walks with us, guiding and protecting us every step of the way. His presence isn't dependent on our circumstances; it's a constant, unchanging reality.

Second, God's presence is rooted in His love. The Bible tells us that God is love, and His love is unconditional and everlasting. In Romans 8:38-39, Paul writes, "I'm absolutely convinced that nothing—nothing living or dead, angelic or demonic, today or tomorrow, high or low, thinkable or unthinkable—absolutely nothing can get between us and God's love because of the way that Jesus our Master has embraced us" (MSG). This passage reassures us that God's love is so strong that nothing can separate us from it. His love for us means that He will never abandon us, no matter what we go through. Even when we feel unworthy or distant from God, His love remains constant. It is this love that drives Him to stay close to us, to never leave us, and to always be by our side.

Third, God's presence is experienced through the Holy Spirit. When Jesus was preparing His disciples for His departure, He promised them a Helper—the Holy Spirit— who would be with them forever. In John 14:16-17, Jesus says, "I will talk to the Father, and he'll provide you another Friend so that you will always have someone with you. This Friend is the Spirit of Truth" (MSG). The Holy Spirit is God's presence within us. He lives in us, guiding, comforting, and empowering us in our daily lives. The Spirit is a constant reminder that we are never alone. Even when we can't see or feel God's presence in a tangible way, the Holy Spirit is there, working in and through us. This is a powerful assurance that God is always with us, not just around us, but within us.

In conclusion, the Bible clearly teaches that God is always with us and will never leave us. This truth is based on His eternal promise, His unbreakable love, and the presence of the Holy Spirit in our lives. No matter what we face, we can hold on to the assurance that God is by our side, guiding us, loving us, and living within us. As we walk through life's challenges, let's remember these reasons and take comfort in the fact that God is always with us, and He will never leave us.

THE PODCAST TRANSCRIPT

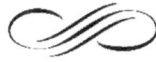

TERENCE: Hey everyone, welcome back. It's good to be with you again as we take another deep dive into the scriptures. And this idea that God is always with us is kind of a basic in our faith, but sometimes we just say the words without really feeling that deep down, you know?

KATIE: Yeah.

TERENCE: So that's what we're digging into today. How can we actually live with that confidence that no matter what God is right there with us?

KATIE: And we're gonna be looking at a passage that really breaks this down into three powerful reasons. It's exciting because it's not just about having some kind of emotional experience, it's about grounding our faith in something solid, something real.

TERENCE: I love that. And you know what else I love about this passage? It doesn't just throw out these vague promises. It gives us an example. It talks about Joshua, you know, Joshua leading the Israelites into the Promised Land. Talk about a high pressure situation.

KATIE: Oh man, can you imagine? I mean, the weight on that guy's shoulders, the uncertainty, the fear of the unknown. And yet, right there in that moment, God gives him this incredible promise. He says, I will be with you. I will never leave you nor forsake you. And it's not just a casual, oh, don't worry. It'll be all right. This is God making a covenant, an unbreakable vow.

TERENCE: So how does that apply to us today? I mean, it's easy to think, well, Joshua is this major biblical figure. God probably made a special exception for him.

KATIE: See, and that's where things get really interesting. When you dig deeper into Joshua's story, you see he faced challenges just like we do, difficult decisions, opposition from enemies, even moments of doubt, right? And what's amazing is that in those very moments, the passage shows us how God's presence wasn't some abstract idea. It manifested in concrete ways. He gave Joshua wisdom, courage, and even supernatural victories.

TERENCE: Gimme an example. What's one way that God showed up so clearly in Joshua's life?

KATIE: Well, think about the battle of Jericho. I mean, the odds were completely stacked against Joshua and the Israelites. No siege weapons, no clear strategy. And what does God tell them to do? March around the city walls for seven days blowing trumpets. Can you imagine having to trust God would come through in such an unconventional way?

TERENCE: I know, right? That takes a whole other level of faith, especially when you're facing something as intimidating as Jericho. So God's promise to Joshua wasn't just, Hey, I'm here. It was, I'm here and I'm gonna show up powerfully in the middle of this battle for you.

KATIE: Exactly. And that's what's so awesome about this promise. Just like with Joshua, it extends to every aspect of our lives, our careers, our relationships, even those internal battles we face within ourselves. You know?

TERENCE: Yeah.

KATIE: He's not just a distant observer. He's actively involved in helping us overcome obstacles and walking victory.

TERENCE: Okay. That is incredible. To think about the same God who fought for Joshua fighting for us today, but the passage doesn't stop there. Right. There's another reason why we can be sure God is with us.

KATIE: Right? The passage goes on to say that God is always with us because he loves us.

TERENCE: Well, yeah, of course. God loves us. But this passage seems to be saying something more like it's not just a general kind of love.

KATIE: Yeah, you're right. It uses the word unconditional, which we hear all the time. But what's the passage really saying about God's love?

TERENCE: That's what I wanna know, because frankly, our human love, it's pretty conditional a lot of the time, isn't it?

KATIE: Absolutely. We tend to love people based on, I don't know, maybe how they make us feel or if they meet our needs, but God's love, it's different. The passage calls it a go love, which is about commitment, a choice. It doesn't come and go based on what we do or don't do. It

TERENCE: Doesn't disappear when we mess up or make bad decisions.

KATIE: It doesn't go away. It's constant, unwavering, even when we don't deserve it, even when we push him away.

TERENCE: Wow. We all need to hear that. But does the passage give any evidence for this?

KATIE: It does. It actually quotes Romans 8.3839, where it says, for I am convinced that neither death nor life, neither angels nor demons, neither the present nor the future, nor any powers, neither height nor depth, nor anything else in all creation, will be able to separate us from the love of God that is in Christ Jesus, our Lord.

TERENCE: Wow. When you put it like that, so like the writer is trying to cover all the bases.

KATIE: Yeah.

TERENCE: Like there's literally nothing that can come between us and God's love.

KATIE: That's exactly it. No matter what you're going through, no matter how far you stray, you can never outrun or escape God's love.

TERENCE: Now, that is a powerful truth.

KATIE: Yeah.

TERENCE: So you've got these two incredible reasons why God is always with us.

KATIE: Yeah.

TERENCE: His promise and his love. But I feel like this passage takes it even one step further, right? This is where it gets really practical, right? This whole idea of the Holy Spirit, like the passage actually calls the Holy Spirit, the third reason why we can be so confident that God is with us always.

KATIE: Yeah. And I think what's really cool is that the passage goes beyond just, you know, talking about the Holy Spirit. It really emphasizes how actively involved the Holy Spirit is in our lives. This isn't just some vague idea of God out there somewhere. This is personal.

TERENCE: So it's not some distant force in the universe, but something much more, I dunno, tangible, more real.

KATIE: Think about it, when Jesus was getting ready to leave his disciples, how did he comfort them? He told them that he wouldn't leave them as orphans. He would send them another helper, an advocate, the Holy Spirit, and get this. He said that the Holy Spirit would be with them. With them forever.

TERENCE: That's right. It's in John, isn't it? He talks about the Holy Spirit, not just being with them, but in them. That always flows me away when I think about it.

KATIE: Totally. It's mind blowing because yeah, it's not just this general idea of God being somewhere out there. It's God himself living and moving within us. In fact, the passage goes on to compare the Holy Spirit to a constant companion, always there providing guidance, offering wisdom and comfort, helping us navigate, you know?

TERENCE: Oh, I love that. That makes it so much more real than just thinking about the Holy Spirit in some kind of theological way, right? It's like having a, I don't know, like having someone walking beside us through the ups and downs of life. Who really gets us, you know better than we even get ourselves.

KATIE: And because the Holy Spirit is God, we have access to all of God's power and guidance whenever we need it.

TERENCE: Man, that is amazing. So bringing this all together, we have these three unbelievable reasons why even when things get really hard, even when we feel alone, God is right there with us. His promise, his crazy, relentless love for us, and the Holy Spirit, our constant companion. And this isn't just some nice idea that makes us feel warm and fuzzy inside. This is the truth that can radically change our lives, right?

KATIE: I think so. You know, for me, what's so beautiful is how these three reasons, the promise, the love, the Holy Spirit, they all weave together because it's God's love that makes him wanna promise these things in the first place. And then it's his love that makes him keep those promises, and it's the Holy Spirit that makes all of that real and powerful in our lives every single day.

TERENCE: This has been so good. I feel like we've gone way past just saying the words, God is with us. We're actually getting a glimpse of what that really means. So as we wrap up today, I want to ask you, what's sticking with you? What really stood out to you? The fact that God actually promises to be with us, or maybe it was a reminder that no matter what His love is always there, or the idea of the Holy Spirit as this constant companion and guide, whatever it is, hold onto it. Let it sink deep into your heart. Because when we truly grasp this truth that God is always with us, it changes everything. It changes how we see ourselves, how we approach our lives, how we face our fears. Until next time, keep seeking, keep exploring and keep driving deeper into the heart of God.

THE STUDY GUIDE

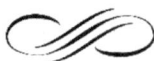

God's Constant Presence

I. Quiz

1. What promise does God make to Joshua, and how does this promise extend to all believers?

2. How does Romans 8:38-39 describe the strength of God's love?

3. What role does the Holy Spirit play in a believer's life according to John 14:16-17?

4. How does the excerpt differentiate between God being "with us" and God being "around us"?

5. What is the main point the excerpt aims to convey to its readers?

6. Identify two challenges or situations where remembering God's constant presence could provide strength.

7. What impact does understanding God's unwavering presence have on a believer's life?

8. How does the excerpt describe the nature of God's love, particularly in relation to human fallibility?

9. Why might understanding the Holy Spirit as God's presence be significant for a believer?

In your own words, summarize the three reasons provided for why God is always with believers.

II. Answer Key

1A. God promises Joshua, "I'll be with you. I won't give up on you; I won't leave you." This promise extends to all believers as a testament to God's unwavering commitment to his people.

2A. Romans 8:38-39 emphasizes the unbreakable nature of God's love, stating that nothing, whether present or future, earthly or spiritual, can separate believers from it.

3A. According to John 14:16-17, the Holy Spirit serves as a constant guide, comforter, and empowerer, representing God's presence within believers.

4A. he excerpt distinguishes "with us" from "around us" by highlighting the Holy Spirit's indwelling, signifying a deeper level of intimacy and connection than mere external presence.

5A. The excerpt aims to reassure believers of God's unwavering presence and encourage them to find comfort and strength in this truth.

6A. Remembering God's presence can provide strength during times of grief, loss, fear, doubt, persecution, or significant life decisions.

7A. Understanding God's constant presence brings peace, courage, and the assurance that believers are never truly alone in their struggles.

8A. The excerpt describes God's love as unconditional and everlasting, remaining constant even when individuals feel unworthy or distant.

9A. Understanding the Holy Spirit as God's presence provides believers with a tangible experience of God's closeness and empowers them to live faithfully.

The three reasons are: God's unchanging promise to be with his people, his unbreakable and unconditional love, and the indwelling presence of the Holy Spirit in believers' lives.

III Essay Questions

1. Analyze the significance of God's promise to be with his people, drawing from both the excerpt and other relevant biblical passages.

2. How does the concept of the Holy Spirit as God's indwelling presence impact a believer's understanding of prayer, worship, and daily living?

3. Discuss the implications of God's unconditional love in light of human failure, doubt, and the challenges of living a faithful life.

4. Compare and contrast the different ways God's presence is experienced and understood throughout the Bible, referencing specific examples.

5. How can the assurance of God's constant presence provide comfort and strength in the face of adversity, uncertainty, and the complexities of the human experience?

IV. Glossary of Key Terms

Holy Spirit: The third person of the Trinity, understood as God's active presence within believers, providing guidance, comfort, and empowerment.

Unconditional Love: Love that is not dependent on any conditions or stipulations, remaining constant regardless of circumstances or behavior.

Indwelling: The concept of God residing within believers through the Holy Spirit, fostering a deep and intimate connection.

Promise: A declaration assuring that something specific will happen, often referring to God's unwavering commitments to his people.

Eternal: Without beginning or end, existing outside the constraints of time, often used to describe God's nature and promises.

FREQUENTLY ASKED QUESTIONS

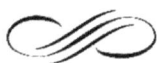

1. Why does God promise to always be with us?

This promise stems from God's very nature and His deep love for His people. It's a testament to His unwavering commitment to guide, protect, and support us throughout our lives, regardless of our circumstances.

2. What is the significance of God's promise to Joshua?

In Joshua 1:5, God reassures Joshua, "I'll be with you. I won't give up on you; I won't leave you." This promise extends beyond Joshua to encompass all believers. It highlights the enduring nature of God's presence, offering comfort and strength in challenging times.

3. How does Romans 8:38-39 illustrate God's constant presence?

This passage emphasizes the strength and constancy of God's love. It states that nothing, regardless of its nature or power, can separate us from His love. This unwavering love ensures He will never abandon us.

4. What role does God's love play in His decision to be with us always?

God's love is the driving force behind His constant presence. His love is unconditional, everlasting, and the very essence of His being. It compels Him to remain close to us, regardless of our actions or feelings of worthiness.

5. How does the Holy Spirit factor into God's promise to never leave us?

The Holy Spirit, as promised by Jesus, serves as God's presence within us. He dwells in believers, offering guidance, comfort, and empowerment in our daily lives. This indwelling presence assures us that we are never truly alone.

6. Can we always feel God's presence in a tangible way?

While we may not always physically feel God's presence, the Holy Spirit serves as a constant reminder of His unwavering closeness. He works within us, even when we are unaware, guiding us and strengthening our connection to God.

7. What is the most comforting takeaway from knowing God is always with us?

The most comforting takeaway is that no matter what challenges, fears, or uncertainties life may bring, we can face them with courage and hope, knowing that God is by our side every step of the way.

8. How can understanding God's constant presence impact our lives?

Recognizing God's unwavering presence can transform our lives by providing peace, strength, and guidance. It fosters a deeper sense of intimacy with God, empowering us to navigate life's complexities with confidence and grace.

CHAPTER FIVE

BELIEF #5

Why God wants you to be happy and healthy and excited about living!

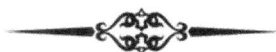

CHAPTER FIVE / BELIEF #5 – TABLE OF CONTENTS

BELIEF #5

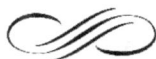

Why God wants you to be happy and healthy and excited about living!

God wants you to be happy, healthy, and excited about living. This truth is woven throughout the Bible, showing that God cares deeply about our well-being. He created us with a purpose and desires that we live fulfilled lives, enjoying the blessings He provides. Let's explore why this is true by looking at some key principles from Scripture.

First, it's important to understand that God's intentions for us have always been good. When God created the world, He made everything with care and love, including us. Genesis tells us that after creating humans, God saw everything He had made, and it was "very good." This shows that from the beginning, God intended for us to live in a world where we could thrive. He didn't create us to be miserable, sick, or weighed down by the burdens of life. Instead, He created us to experience joy, health, and a sense of purpose.

One of the most comforting truths in the Bible is that God delights in our happiness. In Psalm 37:4 (The Message), we read: "Keep company with God, get in on the best. Open up before God, keep nothing back; He'll do whatever needs to be done." This verse encourages us to stay close to God, knowing that He is eager to bless us with what's best for our lives. God knows the desires of our hearts, and when we

91

trust Him, He brings about the kind of joy that is deeper and more lasting than anything the world can offer.

Another essential aspect of God's desire for us to be happy and healthy is the emphasis on the abundant life that Jesus offers. In John 10:10 (The Message), Jesus says, "I came so they can have real and eternal life, more and better life than they ever dreamed of." Jesus didn't come to impose burdens on us but to free us from them. He wants us to experience life to the fullest, not just in eternity but here and now. This abundant life includes spiritual richness, emotional well-being, and physical health. Jesus' ministry on earth was filled with healing, teaching, and acts of compassion, all pointing to God's desire for us to live well.

Living an excited and fulfilled life also ties into the concept of purpose. God has given each of us unique gifts, talents, and opportunities, and He wants us to use them for His glory and our joy. In 1 Peter 4:10 (The Message), it says, "Be generous with the different things God gave you, passing them around so all get in on it: if words, let it be God's words; if help, let it be God's hearty help. That way, God's bright presence will be evident in everything through Jesus, and He'll get all the credit as the One mighty in everything— encores to the end of time. Oh, yes!" When we discover our God-given purpose and live it out, we experience a deep sense of satisfaction and excitement about life. We realize that we are part of something bigger than ourselves, contributing to God's kingdom in a meaningful way.

However, this doesn't mean that life will always be easy or that we won't face challenges. The Bible is clear that difficulties are part of life in a fallen world. But even in the midst of trials, God is with us, working for our good. Romans 8:28 (The Message) reminds us, "That's why we can be so sure that every detail in our lives of love for God is worked into something good." God doesn't abandon us in our struggles. Instead, He uses them to shape us, to make us stronger, and to bring about a deeper joy that isn't dependent on circumstances.

Ultimately, the happiness, health, and excitement God wants for us are found in a relationship with Him. When we walk closely with God, we experience His peace, joy, and love in ways that transform our lives. We learn to trust Him with our worries, to seek His guidance in our decisions, and to find our strength in His presence. This doesn't just make us feel good; it makes us whole. God's plan for us is holistic, touching every aspect of our being—spiritual, emotional, physical, and relational.

In conclusion, God's desire for us to be happy, healthy, and excited about living is rooted in His deep love for us. He created us to thrive, and He has provided everything we need to live abundant lives. By staying close to Him, trusting in His goodness, and living out our purpose, we can experience the fullness of life that God intended. And even when life is hard, we can hold onto the promise that God is working everything together for our good. So, let's embrace the life God has given us, confident that He wants the best for us, and excited about the journey ahead.

THE PODCAST TRANSCRIPT

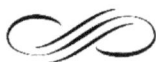

KATIE: Hey everyone. Welcome back. You know, in our last deep dive we got a ton of questions and comments about this whole idea from the text we were looking at that God actually wants us to be happy and healthy, like really wants that for us. Wild.

TERENCE: It is a big counterintuitive, isn't it? Given how much suffering there is in the world.

KATIE: Yeah, exactly. And this deep dive, we're gonna unpack that. We're gonna see what the source has to say about how that's even possible. You know, with all the tough stuff life throws at us,

TERENCE: It'll be interesting to see how this source tackles that tension.

KATIE: Hmm.

TERENCE: Because it's definitely something a lot of people struggle with. Uh,

KATIE: For sure. So to catch everyone up, we're looking at excerpts from this, well it's kind of a devotional, kind of a self-help guide all based on these bible verses about living a full life. And one of the first things that jumped out, at least to me was how it keeps coming back to this idea of God's creation originally being very good.

TERENCE: Right. And that includes us humanity is part of that original goodness. It's not like we were designed for misery from the get go.

KATIE: Exactly. So if things were initially very good, where did it all go wrong? Like how does the source reconcile that starting point with all the very real struggles we face in life?

TERENCE: Well, it doesn't shy away from hardship. It acknowledges that it's part of the human experience, but the source emphasizes that hardship isn't the primary plan. It's more like imagine a beautifully crafted instrument, but someone's playing it out of tune.

KATIE: Okay, I like where you're going with this.

TERENCE: So the potential for beauty is still there. Right. But it's up to us to learn how to play in tune with how we are made. And hardship often comes when we're out of sync with that design.

KATIE: I love that analogy. So aligning with this blueprint for a good life. Okay, I'm hooked. But where do we even begin to understand what that looks like practically?

TERENCE: Well, one of the first places the source points us is towards joy. And it doesn't just say God tolerates our happiness, but that he actually delights in it.

KATIE: Yeah.

TERENCE: Like he genuinely enjoys seeing us joyful.

KATIE: Right. There's that one verse, I think it's in Psalms, delight yourself in the Lord and he will give you the desires of your heart.

TERENCE: Exactly. Psalm 37.4. It's like he's saying, I want you to experience the best life has to offer.

KATIE: That's what gets me that phrasing. It's like picturing someone you love and how their joy brings you joy. This feels similar, but on a cosmic scale, you know,

TERENCE: It's a beautiful way to think about it, but it's important to note the text seems to differentiate between fleeting happiness and a deeper kind of joy tied to our relationship with God.

KATIE: So are we supposed to like swear off all earthly pleasures, be joyful all the time, no matter what, because that seems well impossible. Honestly,

TERENCE: That's a really good point. And it's something that text addresses. It's not about denying ourselves enjoyment. It's more at the why behind

KATIE: It. But why? Okay.

TERENCE: Like imagine two people eating the same delicious meal. One is fully present, grateful, really savoring each bite. The other is scarfing it down, barely tasting it, focused on just getting more. Same act, totally different experience.

KATIE: Oh, I see what you mean.

TERENCE: So it's about cultivating a depth of joy, right. That God can actually delight in seeing that kind of joy that comes from being connected to something bigger than ourselves, not chasing fleeting highs and lows.

KATIE: It's about the source of the joy, not just the joy itself. That's really helpful. So we've got alignment with God leading to deeper joy, which he delights in seeing in us what else is in this blueprint? So it's about the source of the joy, not the joy itself. That's really helpful. So we've got alignment with God leading to deeper joy, which he delights in seeing in us. What else is in this blueprint?

TERENCE: Well, the text goes on to talk about abundant life. And it's interesting because it's not just talking about the afterlife, you know heaven, it's talking about abundant life right here, right now.

KATIE: Okay. That's exciting. But also kind of vague, right? Like what does abundant life actually look like in the day-to-day? Should we all be like living in mansions?

TERENCE: Right? That's a common misconception. And the text is careful not to define abundance in those terms. You know, purely material wealth and possessions. It's not like mansions and sports cars for everyone.

KATIE: Okay, good. Because I can't even afford a new bicycle right now, let alone a mansion.

TERENCE: Yeah. It's definitely not about that. Instead it talks about abundance and encompassing our spiritual, emotional endy, physical wellbeing. This idea of like thriving on multiple levels.

KATIE: I love that it's not just about one area of our lives being good while everything else is falling apart.

TERENCE: Right, exactly. It's about seeking wholeness in every area, even when you know, life throws curve balls,

KATIE: Which it always does. Am I right?

TERENCE: Pretty much. But it made me think of something we were talking about Jesus healing people earlier, which obviously fits with this whole topic. But if we're aiming for this abundant life, does that mean we're meant to be like perfectly healthy all the time? That's something I wrestled with too, honestly. And if you look at the text, it doesn't actually shy away from the reality that we live in a world where well bad things happen.

Sickness, disappointment, suffering, they all exist.

KATIE: So it's not about never experiencing any hardship or health challenges,

TERENCE: Right? It's more about how we respond when those things come up because let's be real, they're gonna come up.

KATIE: So <laugh> we're just supposed to like grin and bear it.

TERENCE: Not exactly. Remember that whole idea of aligning with God's design? It's less about avoiding hardship altogether and more about how we allow those challenges to, I guess, refine us, to draw us closer to God, to deepen our dependence on him. It's about that continuous journey of seeking wholeness even when things get tough.

KATIE: Okay, that makes sense. So instead of striving for a life completely free from pain or problems, it's more about viewing those experiences through the lens of our relationship with God and allowing them to draw us closer to him.

TERENCE: You got it. Think of it like, um, a gardener attending their plants. They can provide water, sunlight, nutrients, the best care in the world, but sometimes a storm rolls in. Right?

KATIE: And that doesn't mean the gardener's a failure.

TERENCE: Exactly. It just means they tend to, the damage help those plants recover and they continue to nurture their growth. This abundant life concept

KATIE: Seems

TERENCE: To suggest a similar posture toward our own lives.

KATIE: That's a really helpful way to look at it. It's about trusting that even when things are hard, God is still present, still working, and still committed to our growth and restoration. So we've got aligning with God's design, leading to deeper joy. We're aiming for abundance in every area of life, even when it's hard. What else is part of this blueprint?

TERENCE: This is where it gets really interesting. The text connects this idea of abundant life to excitement. It basically says that God has given each of us unique talents, passions, gifts, and he wants us to use them. There's that great line in one Peter, I think chapter four, verse 10. It talks about using our gifts to serve others, making God's goodness evident in everything we do.

KATIE: Okay, I remember that one.

TERENCE: Yeah.

KATIE: And it's not just about being like content or at peace, right? It's about being lit up by our lives.

TERENCE: Yeah, exactly.

KATIE: There's this connection the text makes between living out our God-given purpose and feeling genuinely excited to be alive. But how in the world are we supposed to figure out what our purpose actually is? Because it's not like this text comes with, you know, a personalized career aptitude test.

TERENCE: That's the million dollar question, isn't it? It really is. And honestly, it's something a lot of people get stuck on.

KATIE: Totally. It can feel really overwhelming, like what's my purpose? What am I meant to do with my life? Big questions, right?

TERENCE: Sure, sure. But while this text doesn't give us like a step-by-step guide,

KATIE: Yeah,

TERENCE: It does give us some pretty good clues to work with.

KATIE: Okay. I like clues. Lay 'em on me

TERENCE: First. It talks a lot about staying connected to God, like really connected. The source says that through prayer, through really reflecting on scripture, we can start to see where God might be leading us.

KATIE: So it's not necessarily about some big dramatic, you know, burning bush moment

TERENCE: <laugh>. Not necessarily. It could be,

KATIE: Yeah.

TERENCE: But it's more often those little nudges, those moments where you sense God's leading. Maybe it's something you're drawn to, something you're naturally good at. Something that just lights you up inside.

KATIE: Make those aha moments.

TERENCE: Exactly. And a lot of times those aha moments are tied to serving others, making the world a better place in some way. It's like this cool intersection of your passions and God's heart for the world, you know?

KATIE: So it's not like our purpose is this big mystery we have to solve on our own, but something that unfolds as we draw closer to God and you know, pay attention to how he wired us in the first place.

TERENCE: That's it. Exactly. It becomes less about, ugh, I have to figure out my purpose and more about surrendering to who you already are in Christ and then allowing him to use those passions and gifts for something way bigger than yourself.

KATIE: I love that takes the pressure off for sure.

TERENCE: Absolutely.

KATIE: Okay, so we've covered some serious ground here. Aligning with God's design leads to deeper joy, which he loves to see. We're aiming for abundance in every area of life, even when things are tough and through it all, we're discovering and using our God-given gifts to you know, love on others and just make the world a brighter place. That's

TERENCE: A lot. It is a lot. But honestly, I think that's the beauty of this whole blueprint idea, right? It's comprehensive,

KATIE: But there's one more thing we haven't really touched on, and that's just how hard life can be. Even when we are trying to live this way. The text acknowledges that challenges are well inevitable, even when we are walking with God.

TERENCE: It's true. Doesn't sugarcoat that at all,

KATIE: But it doesn't leave us there either. Right?

TERENCE: Right. It actually gives us a super encouraging perspective on challenges. Basically, even when things are tough, even when it hurts, God is still working. He's still there and he's going use those experiences for good. You know that verse from Romans, and we know that in all things, God works for the good of those who love him.

KATIE: Romans 8.2 A is one of my favorites, but also to be honest, one I've wrestled with because if God works everything for good, does that mean we should just like passively accept whatever happens?

TERENCE: That's the question, isn't it?

KATIE: Is it wrong to try to make things better, to change our circumstances?

TERENCE: It's about finding that balance between surrender and action, trusting that God is in control, that he can handle it, but also recognizing that we have a part to play to.

KATIE: So what it's like this ongoing conversation with God like, okay, God, you're clearly working here. What are you trying to teach me through this? And is there anything you're calling me to do about it?

TERENCE: That's a great way to put it. It's a dance, you know? Yeah. Between trusting and doing

KATIE: Reminds me of that quote. Pray like it all depends on God, but work like it all depends on you. This source has that same energy for sure.

TERENCE: Totally. It's this really hopeful, empowering message. We aren't just along for the ride, you know? We're active participants in our own growth.

KATIE: Love that. Well, we have covered so much from aligning with God's design to discovering our unique purpose, navigating challenges. I feel like we could talk about this stuff for days.

TERENCE: We too. It's so rich.

KATIE: As we wrap up here, any final thoughts from the source that really stood out to you?

TERENCE: Honestly, I think the biggest takeaway is this. This source doesn't treat happiness or health or excitement as things we have to achieve on our own. It's not like a to-do list, right?

KATIE: Right.

TERENCE: It's about recognizing that those things are a natural result of aligning our lives with God. When our relationship with him comes first, it's like everything else just falls into place. Which isn't to say life will be perfect or easy or pain free.

KATIE: No, definitely not.

TERENCE: But it does mean that even the hard stuff will have a deeper meaning. A purpose will be able to face it from a different place.

KATIE: Man, that's good. It's not about striving to create a good life for ourselves, but about surrendering to the one who already knows the good life he has planned for us.

TERENCE: Exactly. It's about trust ultimately.

KATIE: I love that. So for everyone listening, here's something to think about as you go about your day. If our lives are meant to be very good, like overflowing with joy and purpose, and yes, even abundance, what might you be overlooking in how you're approaching your own wellbeing? Is there a small shift in perspective, in action that might help you tap into that abundant life a little more fully? Just something to consider. Thank you so much for joining us on this deep dive, everybody. It's been so great unpacking these ideas with you. Until next time, keep seeking. Keep growing and keep living those very good lives. Hmm.

THE STUDY GUIDE

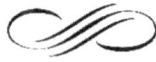

Understanding God's Desire for Our Well-being

I. Short-Answer Quiz

1. According to Genesis, how did God describe His creation, including humanity? What does this reveal about His intentions?

2. Paraphrase Psalm 37:4 and explain its significance in understanding God's desire for our happiness.

3. How does John 10:10 illustrate Jesus's mission and its connection to the abundant life He offers?

4. What connection does 1 Peter 4:10 make between using our God-given gifts and experiencing joy?

5. While affirming God's desire for our happiness, how does the excerpt acknowledge the reality of difficulties in life?

6. According to Romans 8:28, what is God's role in our struggles?

7. Where does the excerpt ultimately locate the source of true happiness, health, and excitement?

8. How does the excerpt describe the nature of God's plan for us in terms of its scope and impact?

9. Summarize the main reasons given for why God desires our happiness, health, and excitement.

10. What call to action does the excerpt conclude with, and what does it encourage readers to embrace?

II. Answer Key

1A. Genesis states that God saw everything He had made, and it was "very good." This shows that God intended for humanity to thrive and experience joy, health, and purpose, not misery or burden.

2A. This verse encourages us to stay close to God and be open with Him. Because He wants what's best for us, He "will do whatever needs to be done" to bless us.

3A. Jesus states that He came so that people can have "real and eternal life, more and better life than they ever dreamed of." This illustrates that His mission was to free us from burdens and empower us to live life to the fullest in the present and future.

4A. The verse encourages generosity with our gifts, using them to serve others and reflect God's presence. This act of living out our purpose allows God's "bright presence" to be evident, leading to a deep sense of satisfaction and excitement.

5A. The excerpt acknowledges that difficulties are inevitable in a "fallen world," suggesting that challenges are a natural part of life despite God's desire for our well-being.

6A. Romans 8:28 emphasizes that God is actively involved in our struggles, working "every detail" for our ultimate good. He doesn't abandon us but uses challenges to shape us and bring about a deeper, more resilient joy.

7A. The excerpt emphasizes that true and lasting happiness, health, and excitement are found in a relationship with God. Through this relationship, we experience His transformative peace, joy, and love.

8A. God's plan is described as "holistic," encompassing every aspect of our being – spiritual, emotional, physical, and relational. It aims to bring wholeness to every dimension of our lives.

9A. God desires our well-being because of His deep love for us. He created us to thrive, provided for abundant living, and remains present in our struggles, working everything for our good.

10A. The excerpt concludes with a call to action, urging readers to embrace life with confidence in God's goodness and excitement for the journey ahead. It encourages living fully, trusting God, and pursuing our purpose.

III. Essay Questions

1. Analyze the excerpt's central argument that God desires our happiness, health, and excitement.

2. What scriptural evidence and theological reasoning support this claim?

3. Explore the relationship between living a "fulfilled life" and discovering one's "God-given purpose" as presented in the excerpt. How does aligning with our purpose contribute to a deeper sense of joy and satisfaction?

4. While affirming God's desire for our well-being, the excerpt acknowledges the reality of challenges and suffering. How can we reconcile the existence of hardship with the belief in a loving God who wants us to be happy?

5. The excerpt emphasizes the "abundant life" that Jesus offers. What does this concept mean in practical terms? How can we actively cultivate and experience this abundance in our daily lives?

6. The excerpt concludes by urging readers to "embrace the life God has given us." In light of the text's message, what does it mean to embrace life fully, and what role do trust and excitement play in this embrace?

IV. Glossary of Key Terms

Abundant Life: A life characterized by spiritual richness, emotional well-being, physical health, and purposeful living, as promised by Jesus.

God-Given Purpose: The unique set of gifts, talents, and opportunities bestowed upon each individual by God to be used for His glory and our joy.

Holistic: Encompassing the whole person; in this context, God's plan addresses every aspect of our being – spiritual, emotional, physical, and relational.

Fallen World: The state of the world after the Fall of Man, characterized by sin, suffering, and separation from God.

Thrive: To flourish, grow vigorously, and experience well-being in all areas of life.

FREQUENTLY ASKED QUESTIONS

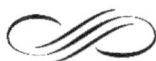

1. Does God really care about my happiness?

Yes! The Bible emphasizes that God delights in our happiness. He created us to experience joy and live fulfilling lives. Psalm 37:4 encourages us to stay close to God, knowing He wants the best for us and is eager to bless us.

2. What does it mean to live an "abundant life" as described in the Bible?

In John 10:10, Jesus speaks of an abundant life, which refers to a life full of spiritual richness, emotional well-being, and physical health. It's a life lived to the fullest, both now and in eternity, free from unnecessary burdens.

3. How does my purpose connect to God's desire for me to be happy?

God has given each of us unique gifts and talents. When we discover and use these gifts for His glory (1 Peter 4:10), we find deep satisfaction and excitement in life, knowing we are part of something larger than ourselves.

4. Does God's desire for my happiness mean I won't face challenges in life?

No, the Bible acknowledges that difficulties are part of life in a fallen world. However, Romans 8:28 reminds us that even in trials, God is with us, working for our good and using those challenges to shape us and deepen our joy.

5. Where can I find true and lasting happiness?

Ultimately, true happiness is found in a relationship with God. When we walk closely with Him, we experience His peace, joy, and love, which transforms our lives and makes us whole.

6. How does God care for my overall well-being?

God's plan for us is holistic. He cares about every aspect of our being—spiritual, emotional, physical, and relational. He desires for us to thrive in all areas of life.

7. What is the first step to experiencing this joy and abundant life God offers?

Begin by nurturing your relationship with God. Trust Him with your worries, seek His guidance in decisions, and find strength in His presence.

8. What is the key takeaway about God's intentions for me?

God deeply loves you and wants you to be happy, healthy, and excited about living. He has created you to thrive, and by staying close to Him, you can experience the fullness of life He intended.

CHAPTER SIX

BELIEF #6

Here is actual proof that God does not want you to be fat, sick, depressed, or unhappy.   How do you know for sure that God has your best interest in mind? Here is proof!

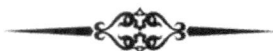

———⟡———

CHAPTER SIX / BELIEF #6 – TABLE OF CONTENTS

BELIEF #6

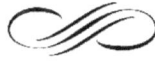

Here is actual proof that God does not want you to be fat, sick, depressed, or unhappy. How do you know for sure that God has your best interest in mind? Here is proof!

God's love and concern for each one of us is woven throughout the entire Bible. He created us, knows us intimately, and desires the very best for us. While life can often present challenges, it's clear from Scripture that God does not want us to be burdened with being fat, sick, depressed, or unhappy. In fact, the Bible offers numerous examples that show how deeply God cares about our physical, emotional, and spiritual well-being. Here is the proof.

First, let's consider the fact that we are created in the image of God. In Genesis 1:27 (The Message), it says, "God created human beings; he created them godlike, reflecting God's nature. He created them male and female." This verse reminds us that we are made in God's likeness, which means our bodies, minds, and spirits are valuable to Him. If we are created to reflect God's nature, it stands to reason that He would want us to be healthy and whole, not weighed down by physical or emotional burdens.

God's desire for our well-being is also evident in the teachings of Jesus. In John 10:10 (The Message), Jesus says, "A thief is only there to steal and kill and destroy. I came so they can have real and eternal life, more and better life than they ever dreamed of." Jesus clearly contrasts His mission with that of the thief—while the enemy seeks to destroy, Jesus came to give us life, and not just any life, but a life that is rich, full, and abundant. This abundant life includes physical health, emotional stability, and spiritual peace. God doesn't want us merely to survive; He wants us to thrive.

Furthermore, we see throughout Scripture that God offers guidance on how to live a healthy and fulfilling life. In 1 Corinthians 6:19-20 (The Message), Paul writes, "Or didn't you realize that your body is a sacred place, the place of the Holy Spirit? Don't you see that you can't live however you please, squandering what God paid such a high price for? The physical part of you is not some piece of property belonging to the spiritual part of you. God owns the whole works. So let people see God in and through your body." Here, Paul emphasizes that our bodies are temples of the Holy Spirit and that we should honor God by taking care of them. This involves making healthy choices in our diet, exercise, and lifestyle. God doesn't want us to be careless with our bodies; instead, He wants us to treat them with respect and care, as they are a precious gift from Him.

But what about our emotional and mental health? God cares about these aspects of our lives as well. In Philippians 4:6-7 (The Message), Paul writes, "Don't fret or worry. Instead of worrying, pray. Let petitions and praises shape your worries into prayers, letting God know your concerns. Before you know it, a sense of God's wholeness, everything coming together for good, will come and settle you down. It's wonderful what happens when Christ displaces worry at the center of your life." God doesn't want us to be weighed down by anxiety, depression, or worry. Instead, He invites us to bring our concerns to Him in prayer, promising that His peace, which transcends understanding, will guard our hearts and minds.

In addition to His concern for our physical and emotional health, God also wants us to experience joy and happiness. In Nehemiah 8:10 (The Message), we read, "He continued, 'Go home and prepare a feast, holiday food and drink; and share it with those who don't have anything: This day is holy to God. Don't feel bad. The joy of God is your strength!'" Here, we see that God's joy is a source of strength for us. He desires for us to experience happiness, not just as a fleeting emotion, but as a deep and abiding state that comes from being in relationship with Him.

In conclusion, the Bible provides clear evidence that God does not want us to be fat, sick, depressed, or unhappy. He created us in His image, sent His Son to give us abundant life, and offers us guidance on how to live in a way that honors Him and promotes our well-being. God's love for us is so great that He desires for us to experience health, peace, and joy in every area of our lives. When we trust in Him and follow His ways, we can be confident that He truly has our best interests in mind. This is the proof that God wants the very best for us, and we can live in the assurance of His love and care each day.

THE PODCAST TRANSCRIPT

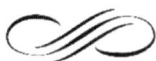

TERENCE: So today we're diving into something that's probably crossed everyone's mind at some point. Does God actually want us to be well, like not just scrape by but truly thrive?

KATIE: The big question for sure,

TERENCE: It really is, and we're gonna dig into it by looking at this excerpt from BIVC Cack six. It lays out this fascinating argument that God actually desires our wellbeing like completely, and the biblical stuff that used to back it up. Surprisingly deep cuts, honestly.

KATIE: Yeah. The source doesn't waste time with the surface level, right from the jump. They go to Genesis 1.27, but, and this is what got me instead of the usual made in God's image, right? They say godlike,

TERENCE: Okay. See that's what I'm talking about. That little language shift, it changes the whole vibe. It's like we're not just cheap knockoffs. There's this potential for real God likeness built into us.

KATIE: And that's the question, right? Yeah. What does that even mean? Godlike? If God is loved, joy, wholeness, all that good stuff, then wouldn't us being Well striving for that. Yeah.

118

Be part of fulfilling that image. It's deeper than just like physical health

TERENCE: Here. It's like imagine looking in a mirror. You don't want that reflection to be all washed out and blurry, do you?

KATIE: Right.

TERENCE: You want to crisp, vibrant. So if we're reflecting the divine in some way, wouldn't that mean God wants us to be well, like in every sense.

KATIE: And the source takes that image even further. Bringing in John 10 point 10 where Jesus talks about more and better life. You know, setting it apart from how the thief operates

TERENCE: And the phrasing not just life, but abundant life. It's like not just existing, but thriving, flourishing. What does that even look like?

KATIE: Yeah,

TERENCE: Practically. You know,

KATIE: It makes you really examine what you value, doesn't it? Because defining abundant life just by stuff, or fleeting pleasure, we're missing something deeper. The text is getting at, it's about purpose, connection, joy, even, which we'll get to wholeness, basically.

TERENCE: Okay. And that brings us to the whole, our bodies are temples thing. Now that gets thrown around a lot, but the source actually

119

unpacks it in one Corinthians 6.19, 20, and they zero in on something most people gloss over. It's not that we have a temple, but that we are the temple.

KATIE: And that changes how you see your whole physical self. If you are sacred space, then taking care of yourself isn't just a chore. It's almost like an act of reverence.

TERENCE: So it's not about following rules to avoid getting in trouble, it's about respecting something valuable. You wouldn't let some historical landmark just crumble, would you?

KATIE: Definitely not.

TERENCE: So how much more care should we take of ourselves if we're walking around in sacred spaces?

KATIE: It's a different way to look at self-care. That's for sure. It's not just like me focused. It's bigger than that. Now, it really makes you think about the whole picture, right? Because we tend to focus on the physical side of being well, but our minds, our emotions, that's all part of it too, isn't it?

TERENCE: Huge. And the source, to their credit, they go there, they bring up Philippians 4.67, you know that whole, don't worry, pray instead bit. But again, they don't just skim the surface. They hone in on how that verse is actually practical advice. It's not about pretending you don't feel worried. It's about putting that energy somewhere else.

KATIE: Shifting the focus.

TERENCE: Exactly. Like instead of getting swallowed by the worry, you connect with something bigger than yourself. That's an active choice, not just wishing the feeling away.

KATIE: And what's really wild is that this ancient wisdom actually lines up with what we know from modern psychology. Like studies show that whether or not you're religious, prayer, meditation, those practices can genuinely reduce stress, good for the mind, good for the body.

TERENCE: So even if you're not totally on board with the whole theological side of it, there's this undeniable link. Our spiritual lives and our mental emotional states, they're intertwined. Makes you wonder, is it just placebo or is there something deeper going on?

KATIE: That's a whole other deep dive right there. But it speaks to how powerful these ancient practices are. They still resonate even with all our modern knowledge. But the source doesn't just stop at worry though. They bring in something we don't always think about in these discussions, joy.

TERENCE: And this is where things get really cool because they point to Nehemiah eight point 10, which links joy with God. Sure. But also with strength. Now we often think of joy as this light, fluffy thing. Maybe even a little frivolous, but strong. That's not a connection you make every day.

KATIE: It challenges the whole idea that joy is somehow less important, less spiritual than things like discipline or perseverance. The source seems to be saying that true joy, the kind that comes from connecting with something bigger than ourselves, that's not just a nice feeling. It's fuel. It gives you strength, helps you face challenges with hope.

TERENCE: It's like instead of joy being this fleeting thing that comes and goes, it's more like this wellspring inside you, this reservoir of strength you can draw on. Even when things are rough, it changes everything.

KATIE: Totally. And it brings us right back to that original point about being made God-Like if God is joy, love, wholeness, then shouldn't we be striving for those things? Wouldn't that be part of fulfilling that image in us?

TERENCE: So it's not just about me and my happiness, it's bigger than that. It's about aligning ourselves with something much greater, something that's always been there. And that's a pretty powerful shift in thinking when you really let it sink in, which makes you wonder, how would it change things if we really believed that? If we stopped thinking we have to earn God's love. Like it depends on us being perfectly healthy and happy all the time.

KATIE: It's a huge weight off your shoulders when you think about it like that. Because what if the source is right? What if our wellbeing, our joy? It's not a condition to be met. It's a reflection of something already there.

TERENCE: So it's less about fixing ourselves up for some divine report card.

KATIE: Yeah.

TERENCE: And more about letting that inherent God likeness shine through.

KATIE: Exactly. And suddenly self-care takes on a whole new meaning. It's not about impressing anyone, it's about stewardship, nurturing that spark within.

TERENCE: And it changes how we see everything, right? Yeah. The choices we make, how we spend our energy, even how we handle those curve balls, life throws at us. 'cause it's not just us trying to muscle through

KATIE: Anymore. There's a deeper well to draw from that strength and joy that comes from being connected to something much bigger than ourselves. It's that abundant life. Jesus talked about, not as some far off reward, but something we can tap into now.

TERENCE: Wow, this deep dive has really taken us place as hasn't it? Ancient texts, modern psychology.

KATIE: Mm-Hmm

TERENCE: <affirmative>. And through it all, this idea that our wellbeing matters more than we realize that it's connected to something almost sacred.

KATIE: It's been quite the journey. And I hope it's just the beginning for our listener.

TERENCE: I do too. So to everyone tuning in, we'll leave you with this. We'll, if taking care of yourself, finding your joy, searching for that peace, what if those aren't just nice to haves, but practices that connect you to something truly profound within What if when you're taking care of yourself, you catch a glimpse of your own God likeness, shining through? Keep those questions alive. Keep exploring, keep diving deep.

KATIE: And until next time, may you find strength and inspiration on your own unique path to wholeness.

THE STUDY GUIDE

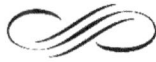

I. Quiz

1. According to the text, how does our creation in God's image relate to his desire for our wellbeing?

2. What contrast does Jesus make between his mission and the actions of a thief?

3. How does 1 Corinthians 6:19-20 explain the importance of caring for our physical health?

4. What guidance does Philippians 4:6-7 offer for dealing with anxiety and worry?

5. According to the text, how is God's joy a source of strength for us?

6. What is the central argument of the excerpt regarding God's desires for humanity?

7. How does the excerpt use the concept of "abundant life" to explain God's intentions?

8. What is the significance of the statement that our bodies are "temples of the Holy Spirit"?

9. How does the excerpt connect our physical, emotional, and spiritual well-being?

10. What action does the excerpt ultimately encourage readers to take in light of God's desires?

II Answer Key

1A. Being created in God's image implies that our bodies, minds, and spirits hold value for him. Therefore, God desires our holistic well-being, reflecting his nature through our health and wholeness.

2A. Jesus contrasts his mission of granting "real and eternal life" with the thief's aim to "steal and kill and destroy." This highlights Jesus's intent to provide a life of abundance, exceeding mere survival.

3A. The passage states that our bodies are "temples of the Holy Spirit," implying a sacred duty to care for them. Honoring God involves making healthy choices in our diet, exercise, and lifestyle.

4A. The passage encourages prayer as a remedy for anxiety and worry. By bringing concerns to God, we invite his peace to displace worry and bring a sense of wholeness.

5A. God's joy is presented as a source of strength, enabling us to experience happiness as a lasting state rooted in our relationship with him. This joy becomes our strength, as seen in Nehemiah 8:10.

6A. The excerpt argues that God desires our complete well-being – physically, emotionally, and spiritually. He doesn't want us to be fat, sick, depressed, or unhappy but to thrive in all aspects of life.

7A. "Abundant life," as mentioned in John 10:10, signifies a life exceeding basic survival. It encompasses physical health, emotional stability, and spiritual peace, showcasing God's desire for us to flourish.

8A. Describing our bodies as "temples of the Holy Spirit" emphasizes their inherent value and sacredness. This concept underscores the importance of treating our bodies with respect and care, reflecting God's presence within us.

9A. The excerpt emphasizes the interconnectedness of our well-being by illustrating how God's care extends to our physical health, emotional stability, and spiritual peace. These elements are not separate but intertwined aspects of a fulfilling life.

10A. The excerpt encourages readers to trust in God and align their lives with his teachings. This trust, coupled with obedience, allows us to experience the fullness of God's love and care in every aspect of our lives.

III. Essay Questions

1. Analyze the excerpt's use of scripture. How do the selected passages support the central claim regarding God's desire for human well-being?

2. Critique the excerpt's interpretation of specific Bible verses. Do you agree with the author's conclusions about God's will regarding health and happiness? Why or why not?

3. The excerpt suggests that God desires our happiness. Discuss the implications of this statement for understanding the nature of God and the purpose of human life.

4. The excerpt emphasizes the connection between physical health and spiritual well-being.

5. Explore this relationship further, considering both the biblical perspective and contemporary perspectives on health and faith.

6. Evaluate the overall effectiveness of the excerpt's argument. Does it convincingly demonstrate God's desire for human well-being? What are its strengths and weaknesses?

IV. Glossary of Key Terms

Abundant life: A life characterized by fullness, richness, and purpose, exceeding mere survival. It encompasses physical health, emotional stability, and spiritual peace, reflecting a life lived in relationship with God.

Temple of the Holy Spirit: A metaphor used to describe the believer's body as the dwelling place of the Holy Spirit. This concept emphasizes the sanctity of the body and the importance of treating it with respect and care.

Wholeness: A state of complete well-being encompassing physical, emotional, and spiritual health. It signifies a harmonious balance in life, reflecting God's design for humanity.

Peace that transcends understanding: A deep and abiding sense of tranquility and serenity that comes from God, surpassing human comprehension. It provides comfort and assurance even amidst challenging circumstances.

Joy of the Lord: A deep and abiding happiness derived from a relationship with God. It is not dependent on external circumstances but flows from an inner wellspring of faith and trust in God.

FREQUENTLY ASKED QUESTIONS

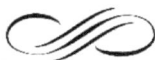

1. Does God care about my physical health?

Yes, the Bible emphasizes that God cares deeply about your physical well-being. You are created in God's image, making your body a temple of the Holy Spirit (Genesis 1:27, 1 Corinthians 6:19-20). Honoring God involves caring for your body through healthy choices in diet, exercise, and lifestyle.

2. Does God want me to be happy?

Absolutely! God desires for you to experience genuine joy and happiness. Nehemiah 8:10 highlights that God's joy is a source of strength, offering a deep and abiding happiness that stems from a relationship with Him.

3. What does the Bible say about God's desire for my overall well-being?

The Bible consistently shows God's desire for your well-being—physically, emotionally, and spiritually. He wants you to thrive, not just survive (John 10:10). This thriving encompasses physical health, emotional stability, and spiritual peace.

4. How does Jesus' mission relate to my well-being?

Jesus' mission directly contrasts the enemy's goal of destruction. He came to give you abundant life—a life richer and fuller than you could imagine. This abundant life includes every aspect of your well-being (John 10:10).

5. Does God care about my mental health?

Yes, God is concerned about your emotional and mental health. Philippians 4:6-7 encourages us to pray instead of worrying, bringing our anxieties and concerns to God. He promises peace that surpasses understanding to guard our hearts and minds.

6. What does it mean to be created in God's image?

Being created in God's image signifies that your body, mind, and spirit hold immense value to Him (Genesis 1:27). It implies that He desires your holistic well-being as a reflection of His nature.

7. How can I be sure God has my best interests at heart?

God's love and concern for you are woven throughout Scripture. He created you, knows you intimately, and desires the best for you. Trusting in Him and aligning your life with His guidance are ways to live in the assurance of His love and care.

8. Does God want me to be overweight, sick, or depressed?

No, the Bible makes it clear that God does not want you to be burdened by illness, depression, or unhappiness. He wants you to experience health, peace, and joy in every aspect of your life. By trusting in Him and following His guidance, you can live a fulfilling life aligned with His best intentions for you.

CHAPTER SEVEN

Is Jesus God?

———❦———

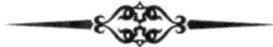

The belief that Jesus is God is central to Christianity. The Nicene Creed (325 AD) states Jesus is "very God of very God" and of the same substance as God the Father. But what does the Bible say? Does Jesus claim to be God?

The Gospel of John opens with: "In the beginning was the Word, and the Word was with God, and the Word was God... The Word became flesh and dwelt among us." This passage shows that Jesus, referred to as "the Word," was with God at creation and is God Himself.

Other biblical passages support this, such as Philippians 2:5-6: "Jesus, being in very nature God, did not consider equality with God something to be used to his advantage." Paul also states in Colossians 2:9-10 that "in Christ, all the fullness of the Deity lives in bodily form."

Jesus makes direct claims to divinity. In John 10:30, He says, "I and the Father are one." In John 8:58, He declares, "Before Abraham was, I am," referring to God's name given in Exodus 3:14, "I Am."

C.S. Lewis argues that Jesus must either be a lunatic, a liar, or truly the Son of God, rejecting the notion that He could be simply a good moral teacher.

The Trinity and the Incarnation.

How can Jesus be both God and man? This is explained through the Trinity: one God in three persons—Father, Son (Jesus), and Holy Spirit. They are distinct, but all are God. The Incarnation refers to God becoming man in the form of Jesus, who, though eternal, took on human flesh to live among us.

Philippians 2:6-8 explains how Jesus humbled Himself to become human and obedient, even to death on the cross, to save humanity.

Why Did God Become Man?

The Incarnation was God's solution to a broken world. Sin separated humanity from God, and no human could fix this. God became man so He could die as a sacrifice for humanity's sins, reconciling us to Him (John 3:16).

St. Athanasius called this the "divine dilemma;" only God could make the perfect sacrifice to restore mankind, and this required Him to take human form.

Salvation Through Jesus.

Jesus' sacrifice offers salvation and eternal life to those who believe in Him. His death and resurrection connect believers back to God, fulfilling the old law.

Romans 5:8 says, "God showed His great love for us by sending Christ to die for us while we were still sinners." Ephesians 2:8-9 emphasizes that salvation is a gift of grace, not something we can earn through good works.

Getting Closer to Jesus.

Living like Jesus, who was fully human AND fully God, means following His example. He knows our struggles and can help us overcome temptation (2 Peter 2:9). He calls us to a relationship with God, offering forgiveness and new life (John 3:3).

Our Jesus Diet is all about living your best life – physically, emotionally, mentally, and spiritually. Jesus wants to transform our spiritual and our physical being. Getting your heart right before God is the most important thing. And then, by fasting and focusing on prayer (an important part of the Jesus Diet and our Membership overall), we can heal physically and spiritually, using that energy for prayer and growing closer to God.

If you haven't already, let Jesus become the light of your world.

The more you move towards the light of Jesus, the less power the darkness will have over you. I hope you can see how this small book can help you focus on the light and not the darkness, no matter where you are on your personal faith journey.

The name "Jesus" literally translates to "God saves!" In the original Hebrew, the name is Yeshua, "salvation," and/or "The Lord who is salvation." It is the name the Angel of the Lord told Joseph to bestow upon Him (Matthew 1:20-21).

There is power in His name: Philippians 2:8-11 says, "Therefore, God also has highly exalted Him and given Him the name which is above every name, that at the name of Jesus every knee should bow, of those in heaven, and of those on earth, and of those under the earth, and that every tongue should confess that Jesus Christ is Lord, to the glory of God the Father."

Through the power of Jesus Christ, you are no longer alienated from God. God is satisfied with the sacrificial death of His son, the perfect lamb, as payment for our sin. He is the completion of the old Law.

In other words... Jesus connects you to God.

Sin is separation from God. It involves pride. It's when we believe that our way is better than God's way. Without Jesus, His sacrifice and resurrection, real connection to God is not possible. We all have sinned. Because of that, we are to be separated from God for eternity. Since God is Holy, there can be no imperfection in His presence.

But all is not lost.

Death was not God's plan for you and me.

Abundant and eternal life (John 10:10) is what Jesus came to bring. We believe that includes your physical, emotional, mental, and spiritual life.

Why? Because even though man was broken and Earth given over to evil, God never stopped loving us. Romans 5:8 says, "But God showed His great love for us by sending Christ to die for us while we were still sinners."

Salvation is when you reconnect to God.

Nothing but Jesus could have fixed the problem. Your best work just can't get you to Heaven. Even if you could somehow achieve a score of 99 out of 100 in life, you'd still need a sacrificial savior to make up the difference and pay off your debt. That's the difference between Grace and the Law. James 2:10 says, "For whoever keeps the whole law and yet stumbles in one point, he has become guilty of all." OUCH!

However, "God saved you by His special favor when you believed. And you can't take credit for this; it is a gift from God. Salvation is not a reward for the good things we have done, so none of us can boast about it." (Ephesians 2:8-9, NLT). You can't earn a gift – it's an unmerited favor.

You do, however, have to make the choice to accept it.

So, as sinners, we all must turn to God for forgiveness of sin, and trust that Jesus died to give us new life that we may be "born again." (John 3:3; 1 Peter 1:23).

Faith is the key. It's the cause and effect of our hope for salvation. If there is truly "no other name under heaven that has been given among men, by which we must be saved" (Acts 4:12), then your acceptance of God's gift, your admission that you are a sinner, your repentance (changing mind), and your faith in the real-but-unseen Lord is all that can bring eternal and abundant life.

Please do this now, before we wrap up this book: If knowing about Jesus has stirred your heart to hear even more, receive forgiveness for your sins, renew your Christian walk, or get involved in ministry, you may pray the following prayer right now, before we wrap up this book...

"Lord Jesus, I know that I am a sinner and ask for your forgiveness. Please come into my heart as my Lord and Savior. Take complete control of my life and help me to walk in Your footsteps daily by the power of the Holy Spirit. Thank you Lord for saving me and for answering my prayer."

When you pray those words deeply and sincerely, I believe you have been born again. You are a new creation, that's what the Bible says. Now you can begin to let Jesus be the light of your world.

Continue to study His Word. Focus on His core teachings I have shared with you in this book and other resources. Begin to study the Bible for yourself. I recommend starting with the Gospels of Matthew, Mark, Luke, and John. And find other like-minded believers you can associate with.

Ok, this would be an good place to wrap up our time together. I hope and pray that you will study this book, refer to it often.

Make The Jesus Diet a part of your life!

I know the focus of this particular book is on the core beliefs we've explored together. But you've heard references to the Jesus Diet, because I believe it really is the best way to achieve optimal health, both physically and spiritually.

Eating food all day and night is bad for your health. You never give your digestive system time to rest, relax, and heal. The Jesus Diet changes all that. It helps your body heal.

When there is no food to digest, your body needs less energy to carry out the other functions. Now that energy can go into physical and spiritual healing. This diet can do that for you.

But that's not all. This diet helps you lose weight and feel better, yes. But it also helps you get closer to Jesus. You can lose or maintain your weight, have more energy and vitality. And it may even help you live longer and avoid certain diseases. But getting closer to Jesus is always the best reason.

It's simple. It's proven. And it's guaranteed to let you lose weight and keep it off. Remember, all I do is wait as long as possible to start eating and then stop as early as possible. I give myself a little bit of leniency because none of us are robots. I try to go through 18 hours of not eating and 6 hours of eating. Follow this simple plan, and the 3 to 5 hours of hunger you experience each day is a small price to pay for all the fantastic life-changing benefits you can achieve. I will teach you a powerful method to deal with the pain of hunger. This is short-term pain to get the long-term gain that can change your life.

This beats all other weight-loss options.

Daily fasting focuses on when you eat, not what you eat. No more counting calories. No more cutting out the foods you love. No more guilt! All you must do is get through the 3 to 5 hours a day when you feel the actual pain of hunger.

We focus on the hunger you feel when you're on this diet. This is the part that most people try to avoid. They don't like to feel hungry. But as you'll see, the small amount of pain from daily hunger can be a positive thing. It can make you feel alive!

The pain I go through on this diet has never been a problem. Why? Because I've discovered a simple 3-step technique to overcome all of life's challenges. I call it the Miracle Method because, like this diet, it can create a miracle in your life.

The uncomfortable feelings of hunger only lasts for a few hours a day. It's something I will help you overcome. That's where my little-known method comes in. I discovered this method many years ago while going through extremely difficult personal problems. It's a method that helps you cope with all kinds of pain, including the small block of time you will feel intense hunger pains on this diet.

Most people don't stay on this diet because of these intense feeling of hunger. They try this diet (because it's so simple), but they feel they can't endure the pain. Some of my students feel as if they will die! They have never felt this kind of hunger, and after a few days (or even one day), they shout, "I CAN'T DO IT!" and they quit. This stops them from losing weight and keeping it off. It also prevents them from getting all the other long-term health benefits of daily fasting...

But the pain of hunger will never be a problem for you.

The main reason you haven't heard about daily fasting is the fact that nobody makes money by telling you not to eat their products, not take their supplements, or not buy their products or services. In other words, fasting is not a very marketable topic, so you're not exposed to advertising and marketing about it.

The result is that it seems somewhat extreme or strange, even though it's not.

Fasting has been around for centuries. Medical practitioners have also noted the health benefits of fasting for thousands of years. In other words, daily fasting isn't some new fad or a crazy marketing ploy. It's been here for a long time, and it works.

But as you also know, most people try this diet for a few days or a week and say: "I have never felt this hungry!" or "I feel like I will starve to death!" or "I have never felt hunger this intense!" or "There's no way I can torture myself like this!" Or the best statement I have read so far...

"I'd rather die than be on this diet!"

This is the language of emotion. They're the kind of words that my students will write down when they use the first step of the Miracle Method. I am excited to show you how this works! Some people feel they're going to die. BUT FEELINGS LIE. That's what the Miracle Method helps you realize. And even though you feel that you may not be able to withstand the short periods of intense hunger...

YOU ARE WRONG!

People have been fasting for centuries. Your body is built to go without food for long periods. The physical pain of hunger comes and goes. You learn to live with the pain of hunger and even learn how to enjoy it. As you'll see, the Miracle Method will teach you how to turn that pain into power!

The 3-step Miracle Method lets you transform your hunger pain into an entirely different experience. This is a spiritual method that lets you make Jesus your partner and let Him remove whatever pain you're suffering from. It can also help you with the short periods of intense feelings of pain you'll experience on this diet. Follow this method, and you'll develop the ability to deal with the few hours of daily hunger, turn your body into a fat-burning furnace and get closer to Jesus. This is a diet that Jesus would want you to be on and the Miracle Method is a 3-step method that will bring you closer to Him.

In Conclusion.

Before you go, I'd like to invite you to become a Member of the Jesus Diet community. You can read about the Jesus Diet in our 300-page book. But Membership is designed to help you get and stay on this amazing life-changing diet. Plus you'll get even more helpful resources like this book, others in this important series, as well as other resources designed to enhance your faith. Read the last page. Become a Member and you'll be on your way to letting Jesus Christ help you transform your health and your life.

141

Jesus' identity as both God and man is foundational to Christian belief. His life, death, and resurrection offer the way to eternal life and reconnection with God. Through fasting (the Jesus Diet or other types of fasting), prayer, and focusing on His teachings, believers can grow in their relationship with Jesus.

A PERSONAL INVITATION

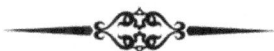

I hope you have enjoyed this book. I initially began writing for this series because of my work with the Jesus Diet. It was an attempt to flesh out some of the ideas we've been working on related to the Jesus Diet, including how this diet can help you lose weight, look great, and increase your faith on your spiritual journey.

If these ideas sound interesting to you, I'd like to personally invite you to check out my 293-page Jesus Diet book. The Jesus Diet book has 12 Chapters:

Ch.1 – What would Jesus Want You to Eat.

Ch.2 – How the Miracle Method Helps You Stay On This Diet.

Ch.3 – 28 Shocking Facts About What's Killing You and the People You Love.

Ch.4 – Why a Gluten-Free Diet Could Save Your Life.

Ch.5 – Why People Are Dying from Avoidable Diseases Caused by Obesity, Such as Diabetes, Heart Disease, and Cancer... and How You Can Avoid Being One of Them.

Ch.6 – Why the Government's "Food Pyramid" Should Be Called the "Food Tombstone."

Ch.7 – The Little-Known Health Benefits of Better Sleep.

Ch.8 – The True Cause of the #1 Killer... and How You Can Avoid It.

Ch.9 – Death Starts in Your Gut.

Ch.10 – The Easy and Fun 30-Minute Cure for Your Biggest Health Problem.

Ch.11 – Here Are 76 Ways That Sugar Can Ruin Your Health.

Ch.12 – Is Jesus God?

You'll definitely want to learn more about how the Jesus Diet and our Miracle Method, along with other key components of the Jesus Diet help you achieve total physical, mental, and spiritual health and wellness. Chapter 2 of the big book, in particular, reveals the Miracle Method; a 3-step process that is the secret to staying on the Jesus Diet and achieving the better life you're aiming for.

Here's how to get your copy of the 293-Page Jesus Diet book and a free 3-month subscription to our Jesus Diet Challenge Newsletter.

1. **Order a copy of our 293-page book, The Jesus Diet.** On the next page, you'll find an Order Form. Fill out the Form and send it to me to receive a copy of The Jesus Diet. It's also available through bookstores everywhere, but you won't get 3 free gifts worth $234. Plus, I'll add you to my list of subscribers to my Jesus Diet Challenge Newsletter for 3 months.

2. **Let me send you <u>3 free months</u> of my Jesus Diet Challenge Newsletter – even if you don't get the big**

book. Even if you don't want to purchase a copy of our big book, The Jesus Diet, you can still claim a 3-month complimentary subscription to our Jesus Diet Challenge Newsletter. It's packed with helpful information about the Jesus Diet, our Miracle Method, and everything else we've discussed in this small book. You'll love it!

Don't miss out on the opportunity to transform your physical and spiritual health and wellbeing. Take action now to continue your journey with the Jesus Diet!

Jesus Diet 293-Page Book and Free Newsletter Order Form

YES, T.J.! I read your book and I'm ready to dive in deeper. Please send me a copy of your big Jesus Diet book and a 3-month subscription to your Jesus Diet Challenge Newsletter. You have proven to me that this diet is something unique and special. I must know more! The book is just $25 (free s/h) and includes your newsletter for 3 months. Or, if I'm not ready to buy the book today, I can start with a free 3-month subscription to your Jesus Diet Challenge Newsletter. Either way, you'll also include the valuable free gifts worth $234 with my first package. *So on that basis, sign me up!*

STEP #1: Choose your option.

❐ **Send me the FREE Jesus Diet Challenge Newsletter (a $37.25 value)!** You'll learn more about the Jesus Diet and Miracle Method over the next 3 months. There's no obligation to purchase the book or become a Member. **SEND NO MONEY!** Enjoy this 3-month subscription as our gift to you.

❐ **Send your Newsletter and 293-Page Book!** Enclosed is **$25**.

STEP #2: Provide your payment information.

Card Number _____ Expiration _____

Signature _____ Security Code _____

STEP #3: Give us your complete contact information.

Name _____ Address _____

City/State/Zip Code _____

Daytime Phone Number _____

Email Address _____

INSTRUCTIONS: Fill out this Form and MAIL or FAX it directly to us.

MAIL to: Jesus Diet/DRN • P.O. Box 198 • Goessel, KS 67053

Or FAX to: (316) 333-1941

Submitting this Form constitutes an acceptance of the terms on the back.

For Internal Use Only:
_____
Referral ID Number

147

www.ingramcontent.com/pod-product-compliance
Lightning Source LLC
Chambersburg PA
CBHW022337280326
41934CB00006B/671